Contents

Deadly Diabetes Lies

DEADLY DIABETES LIES

So exactly what is the Diabetes Industry *not* telling you about diabetes, or should I say how are they misleading you? Let me count the ways...

Lie #1: *"We're not exactly sure what causes prediabetes and type 2 diabetes."* Some experts attribute it to obesity. Others say it's our abysmal modern diet and sedentary lifestyle. Still others blame the patients themselves, implying they are lazy and undisciplined. Rarely does the current medical system place the responsibility where it deserves to be: On the foods you've been taught to crave and believe are safe and healthful. What you're not being told is how terrible they are for your health and how they constitute a *causal link* to this terrible disease.

The Truth: The global pandemic of type 2 diabetes and prediabetes is caused *directly* by our modern diet of highly processed foods. These include high-carbohydrate/low-nutrient junk "foods" and fast food...overly processed refined carbohydrates...and metabolism-distressing ingredients such as sugar and artificial sweeteners...high-fructose corn syrup...trans fats...and refined vegetable oils. Factor in hidden allergies to wheat and other substances (which stress and weaken the immune system) and a catastrophic absence of fiber-rich, nutrient-dense whole foods—including fresh fruits and vegetables, whole grains and beans, and humanely raised, hormone-free meat, eggs, fish, and dairy products—and you have a perfect recipe for diabetes.

The Reason: If this truth were widely revealed, and if public health officials openly condemned this diabetes-causing diet, the economic repercussions would be devastating for the giant agribusiness corporations that grow the raw materials for these commercial "food products," a term I prefer because much of what's produced doesn't qualify as real food for me.

The truth would also hit the manufacturers and marketers who stock these products in our supermarkets; the supermarkets themselves; and the media, which thrive on the advertising revenue these products generate. I assure you that unimaginable sums of money are being generated as diabetes develops and spreads.

Were the medical community to point a finger directly at the foods and beverages causing today's tsunami of type 2 and prediabetes in unaware adults and defenseless children, it would trigger a massive cry from the billion-dollar industries involved—plus a lobbying barrage more colossal than Washington and other capitals around the world have ever seen.

Placing the blame on obesity, lack of exercise or the patients themselves is a deceitful distraction from the true cause. That the medical and scientific communities are complicit in this deceit—or remain silent—borders on malpractice.

Lie #2: *"The American diet (like our medical system) is the best in the world."* We've been conditioned to believe our supermarkets and dinner tables are the envy of the world. And that our doctors and hospitals are the best on the planet.

The Truth: All our food-related government watchdog agencies, which are supposed to be protecting our health, are obstructed by contradictory goals and objectives, as well as by massive special-interest lobbying. This includes the USDA (safety of agricultural products), the FDA (effectiveness and safety of pharmaceutical drugs), the EPA (environmental quality) and the FTC (quality of broadcast programming and advertising). Literally billions of our tax dollars in the form of federal agriculture subsidies are pumped into price supports for sugar, corn, wheat, soybeans and feedlot beef—the raw materials from which many diabetes-causing food products are made. Almost nothing goes to small farmers struggling to raise organic fruits, vegetables, and livestock.

US agricultural capacity, which politicians love to boast about, is based on *volume*, not quality. In actual fact, America's bountiful harvests are the result of copious applications of synthetic fertilizers, herbicides, pesticides, growth hormones, antibiotics and a host of other dubious chemicals that are linked to numerous health problems in our population. Many studies show that these agricultural chemicals depress the body's immune system, compromise the liver (our most important organ for detoxification), and attack the beta cells of the pancreas (which produce insulin). These facts are well known but the scientific community overall remains hauntingly silent. Just one example: 83 active pesticide ingredients known and shown to cause cancer in animals or humans are still in use today.

The Reason: Cleaning up our agricultural system would result in hundreds of billions of dollars in lost profits for every industry involved. As for the superlative quality of our food and medical systems, both are misconceptions. The US is 33rd out of 195 nations in infant mortality, 47th in life expectancy of 226 countries and 13th in heart disease mortality. It is the 16th highest in the incidence of breast cancer, ninth in cancer deaths, and we have nearly four times the incidence of diabetes compared with the world average. When it comes to the incidence of preventable diseases US is 17th in the world, right behind Portugal (number 16); which means it's healthier there than it is here. The one health statistic that we *do* lead every other nation on earth in? *Obesity.*

Lie #3: *"Type 1 diabetes is a genetic phenomenon and there isn't much we can do about it."* The mainstream belief is that type 1 diabetes is an autoimmune disease in which the body's immune system destroys its own insulin-producing beta cells. Once the cells are wiped out, doctors say, they're gone forever and the patient must rely on lifelong insulin injections.

The Truth: Fascinating new research is questioning this belief. For one thing, type 1 diabetes is rapidly rising right along with type 2. Relatively rare 200 years ago, type 1 is now twice as common among children as it was in the 1980s and five times greater than just after World War

II. Epidemiologists say the incidence of type 1 diabetes is 1000% higher than it was 100 years ago.

How can this be true if genetics are responsible? Human genes don't change that rapidly, but our lifestyle and environment certainly have. One emerging theory is that type 1 isn't an autoimmune malfunction at all, but rather the immune system disposing of beta cells that have been damaged in some way—by a virus, environmental toxins or food chemicals, including *alloxan* in white flour and bread.

Research is also disproving the "once they're gone, they're gone" theory about beta cells. Preliminary studies show that certain foods and supplements may indeed regenerate beta cells in the pancreas so they can produce insulin again. Other nutrients have been found to strengthen the remaining beta cells in individuals with type 2 diabetes so that they can once again produce insulin naturally.

Finally, simple lifestyle modifications described in *The 30-Day Diabetes Cure* can increase the body's insulin sensitivity, allowing type 1 patients to dramatically reduce their insulin dosage. My type 1 diabetes patient Jay F. is a good example. He was able to cut his dose by 80% by following *The 30-Day Diabetes Cure*. Insulin reductions like these allow patients to avoid diabetic complications later in life.

The Reason: Call me cynical, but I'm not seeing very much mainstream curiosity about reviving the strength of beta cells—or about getting type 1 patients to lower their doses of insulin (even though this could greatly improve their outcomes). The global insulin market is currently worth $3 billion and growing at 14% annually. Need I say more?

THE BIGGEST LIE OF THEM ALL

Lie #4: *"You can't really cure type 2 diabetes."* This is the biggest lie of them all—and the most damaging. Why? Because it keeps patients powerless and dependent on the Diabetes Industry. It turns them into cash cows to be regularly "milked" by this $400 billion system, even as the purveyors of junky, diabetes-causing food products continue to create more patients for it.

The Truth: Plenty of scientific research proves that both prediabetes and type 2 can be reversed with a few simple diet and lifestyle modifications, just like those presented in *The 30-Day Diabetes Cure*. For example...

■ In 1982, nutritional researcher Kerin O'Dea restored a group of severely diabetic Australian aboriginal men to good health simply by getting them off the typical Western diet of refined carbohydrates and its accompanying sedentary lifestyle (the two major causes of type 2). Not a drop of medication or insulin was required.

5

The men were badly overweight and insulin-resistant, with seriously elevated cholesterol, triglycerides and high blood pressure (all major risk factors for heart attack and stroke). They were headed for a shortened lifespan with miserable complications, including gangrene, blindness, heart failure, various cancers and amputations of digits and limbs caused by nerve damage.

After just seven weeks on her plan, O'Dea drew blood samples and discovered these dramatic changes…

■ Blood triglycerides, glucose and cholesterol levels had plummeted into the healthy range.

■ Blood pressure had dropped significantly and normalized.

■ The men had lost an average of nearly 20 pounds each.

In O'Dea's own words, "All of the metabolic abnormalities of type 2 diabetes were either greatly improved or completely normalized." The markers for diabetes and heart disease were completely gone!

This discovery, in my view, was as significant as some of the most famous in medical history, ranking right up there with Lister (sterilization), Pasteur (germ theory), Fleming (antibiotics), and other medical super-heroes. Like the work of these brilliant earlier medical pioneers, O'Dea's discovery could have prevented unnecessary suffering and saved millions of lives had it been heeded and adopted in mainstream practice. Instead, her research got buried because of medical politics and food industry pressure.

Other research has confirmed O'Dea's finding regarding the prevention and reversal of type 2 and prediabetes, notably…

■ In 1984, the journal *Diabetes* reported on a clinical study done at the University of Vermont College of Medicine proving that increased physical activity boosts cell sensitivity to insulin—thus reversing the insulin resistance that is the precursor to (and underlying cause of) type 2 diabetes. These findings were confirmed by a 2003 study published in *Diabetes Care* demonstrating that sedentary adults who simply added walking to their daily routine cut their risk of developing insulin resistance (prediabetes), *even if they didn't lose any weight*.

■ Researchers at the UCLA School of Medicine found that 50% of type 2 patients were able to *reverse* their diabetes in just three weeks by making small changes in their diet and adding moderate exercise. "The study shows, contrary to common belief, that type 2 diabetes and metabolic syndrome can be reversed solely through lifestyle changes," according to lead researcher Dr. Christian K. Roberts.

■ In 2001, the *New England Journal of Medicine* published research showing that even the simplest dietary changes can reduce the risk of developing type 2 diabetes by nearly 60%. Subsequent studies (which included switching to the delicious, healthful foods you'll discover in *The 30-Day Diabetes Cure*...see also page 63 of this publication) improved this reduction in diabetes to greater than 95%.

- In 2001, the largest study ever conducted to test the ability of diet and exercise to prevent prediabetes from turning into full-blown type 2 proved to be a smashing success. Doctors at 27 medical centers around the country enrolled 3,234 people and assigned them to receive the drug metformin (Glucophage), a placebo or a lifestyle program involving classes and coaches who kept track of their progress. After three years, the lifestyle program cut the participants' risk of developing diabetes by more than 50%—a much better result than metformin provided. "I don't see this as out of reach for the 10 million people who are at high risk for diabetes," said the study's director. (That figure today is closer to 60 million Americans alone.)

- A Duke University Medical School study found that type 2 diabetics who reduced their consumption of carbohydrates achieved better blood sugar control and more effective weight loss than those who went on a typical calorie-restricted diet. After just six months, the low-carb group had lower hemoglobin A1C results, lost more weight with *95% of the participants being able to reduce or even completely eliminate their diabetes medications.* Plus, as little as a five percent weight loss—about 10 pounds for most people in the study—reduced the risk of diabetes by 58%. That is truly remarkable.

"It's simple," says Eric Westman, MD, director of Duke's Lifestyle Medicine Program and lead author of the study. "If you cut out the carbohydrates, your blood sugar goes down, and you lose weight, which lowers your blood sugar even further. It's a one-two punch."

The Reason: By the end of this decade, the Diabetes Industry will be a trillion-dollar business. That's a lot of glucose monitors...test strips...lab tests...doctors visits...drugs and insulin...plus medical supplies and procedures. The scandalous reason there isn't a concerted effort to eradicate diabetes through patient education and public awareness is because there's more money to be made from *treating* it. Curing diabetes just isn't cost effective.

I realize there are many well-intentioned physicians who really care about their patients' well-being. But the current medical system isn't set up to educate and monitor diabetes patients in changing their lifestyle. Health providers won't reimburse doctors for it—in today's overworked physician just doesn't have the time.

A more serious problem is that many conventional physicians have lost faith in the body's remarkable ability to heal and repair itself.

Once upon a time, medicine was an art and physicians were true healers. They knew the incredible power of regeneration that resides within the human body. More important, they were wise enough to respect it. Today, the insurance industry essentially forces doctors to follow "cookbook-type treatments"—and those "recipes" contain plenty of drugs because Big Pharma is creating the menu.

The huge corporations that now control our health care industry (and, therefore, our doctors) have little or no interest in any treatment that can't produce profits for them. Tragically, modern doctors have traveled dangerously far from the spirit of the Hippocratic Oath, which they are sworn to uphold.

Because corporate interests have turned the practice of medicine into a business, many doctors today—even those with the best intentions—simply don't have the time, resources or knowledge to actually *cure* their patients. The best they are allowed or equipped to do is simply manage symptoms.

Yet there are many exciting new health and healing discoveries being made *outside* the realm of conventional medicine that all healthcare practitioners need to open their minds and become "good students" in order to become competent teachers for their patients. In my view, education is the very best medicine—and *The 30-Day Diabetes Cure* packs plenty of it.

Diabetes Lie #5: *"If you have diabetes, it's your own fault."* This is blaming the victim for the disease—and it's shameful.

The Truth: Powerful forces are at work in our culture to encourage poor eating choices and a sedentary lifestyle, beginning at a very early age. Saturday morning and after-school TV is packed with seductive advertisements for diabetes-encouraging foods. We develop these habits, appetites, cravings and brand loyalties at a very early age. Who is there to protect us and our children from these unhealthy products with their billion-dollar marketing budgets? The ADA? The AMA? The FTC? The FDA? The USDA? The PTA? *Hardly.*

LET'S START PLACING THE BLAME WHERE IT'S DESERVED

This area may be where the playing field is most uneven. Blaming the diabetes patient for a "lack of willpower" is like telling people who live near a pollutant-spewing factory not to breathe the air, says Yale's Kelly D. Brownell, PhD, director of its Rudd Center for Food Policy and Obesity.

Most of us believe we're too smart to be influenced by advertising, marketing campaigns, colorful store displays and the sneaky psychological strategies that food marketers employ to push their products on us subconsciously. But, in truth, most consumers are no match for these highly paid masters of manipulation.

IT'S TIME FOR DOCTORS AND HEALTH EDUCATORS TO SPEAK OUT

Just as the public health community once played a central role in wiping out communicable diseases, it now needs to become active in protecting the air we breathe, the water we drink and the food we eat. If it doesn't speak out—and soon!—today's chronic and degenerative diseases will destroy our health, our economy and our society.

Food lobbyists have far too much influence over public health practices and policy. Just like the industries that pollute our air and waterways, manufacturers of unhealthy food products do not pay for the devastating consequences their products wreak upon society. We, the taxpayers, foot those bills; and this is, in effect, a secret subsidy to these industries. This must cease. It is only fair that the price of their unhealthy products include cleaning up the damage they do.

If we ever hope to end the scourge of diabetes, their free ride must come to an end.

...AND IT'S TIME TO STOP BELIEVING THESE DIABETES LIES

We've lost considerable control over our lives in the past decade or two. The power of corporations today reminds me of medieval royalty, which ruled over enslaved serfs who were overtaxed, overworked, and overwrought.

Modern corporatism now controls all of life's essentials, including our access to food, water, medicine, information, energy, and travel—even the air we breathe. We have become "consumers" in every sense of the word with little say and few alternatives.

The one area where we still have a chance to take back our power is our personal health. This requires that we refuse to be milked as a "cash cow" by the Diabetes Industry any longer. This is where we must make our stand.

I wrote *The 30-Day Diabetes Cure* to serve as a step-by-step roadmap for escaping the food and medical industries—and to declare your independence and freedom from them. I'm convinced that these all-too-mighty corporations care more about their bottom lines than your health or well-being. It is a dangerous situation when profits are linked to disease because more disease will be the inevitable outcome

Mistakes Doctors Are Making With Diabetes

MISTAKES DOCTORS ARE MAKING WITH DIABETES

"The part can never be well unless the whole is well."

—PLATO

DESPITE THE HYSTERIA being generated by the medical community and the media, type 2 diabetes and prediabetes are not typical "medical" problems.

Rather, both are *lifestyle* conditions caused by chronic inactivity and unhealthy food choices. As such, they can have a very simple, non-medical, inexpensive and immediate lifestyle solution: Making smarter food and activity choices will usually return the body's glucose metabolism to normal without the need for glucose-lowering medications.

Numerous studies confirm this. Tens of thousands of people diagnosed with diabetes have been able to *completely reverse* their condition and discontinue their medication without having to become a vegetarian (unless they choose to)…without dieting to lose weight…and without exercising like a hamster on a wheel.

Perhaps you're wondering: "If it's so simple, why are so many people still suffering and dying from diabetes and its complications?"

The answer is simple, albeit incredulous: Very little money and effort are going into promoting this lifestyle approach. Instead, diabetes has been "medicalized"—and much to the financial benefit of everyone in the Diabetes Industry, including those profiting from the sale of diabetic supplies, pharmacy sales, hospitals stays, diagnostic tests, doctor visits, and new "diabetes-friendly" food products.

THE CURE NO ONE'S ALLOWED TO TALK ABOUT

Less than one percent of the annual $400 billion currently spent on diabetes globally goes for prevention and patient education. This is difficult to reconcile given that numerous studies clearly show that prevention and education are the most effective tools we have for defeating chronic illness and disease. Look at the huge impact that public awareness campaigns had on cigarette smoking and reducing the spread of HIV/AIDS. There's no reason why today's diabetes pandemic couldn't be halted in its tracks with a similar, all-out campaign. Yet these formidable weapons are *not* being used. And I believe the underlying reason is…

13

THERE'S MORE MONEY TO BE MADE FROM
TREATING DIABETES THAN CURING IT

This is an economic reality. But it's bad news for patients because it shows just how stacked *against* you the deck is. With so many vested interests pushing for the continued medicalization of diabetes, it seems unlikely that the truth may ever emerge in any significant way. You're fortunate that *The 30-Day Diabetes Cure* has found its way into your hands.

It's also unlikely that the many mistakes doctors are currently making in treating diabetes will be exposed in a meaningful way. As a result, you can expect the incidence of this debilitating disease and its severe complications to keep mounting.

I firmly believe we'll never eradicate diabetes until we publicize its dietary causes—and create public awareness that results in people abstaining from these troubling foods and beverages because they are educated about the consequences. In lieu of this, we will continue to be distracted and tantalized by a hopeful quest for an ever-elusive medical cure, instead of popularizing the proven solution we already have: Diet and lifestyle modifications. Meanwhile (and tragically so), millions of people will continue to die from a lifestyle condition that is utterly preventable and reversible.

SERIOUS MISTAKES DOCTORS ARE MAKING WITH DIABETES

Conventional medicine's failure to contain the growth of diabetes and its deadly complications is evident by their dismal statistics. Not only is Big Medicine's overall diabetes strategy ineffective and misguided, but current treatment protocols and drugs actually can *increase* a patient's risk of heart attack and other serious complications. Here's where I believe current medical treatments are erring…

Diabetes Mistake #1: *"Monitoring blood sugar is helpful and necessary for people with type 2 diabetes."* Doctors are fixated on lowering numbers, including glucose levels, triglycerides, cholesterol, or blood pressure—instead of reversing the underlying cause of type 2 and prediabetes, which is insulin resistance. Some insurance companies actually pay doctors bonuses when their diabetic patients drive down their numbers to very low levels.

But this "numbers mentality" leads patients to believe that they can eat whatever they want as long as they just take a pill or inject a little extra insulin to keep their glucose in the normal range. *This is a big mistake.*

In fact, studies show that glucose monitoring is of little to no benefit for type 2 diabetics—and is a needless nuisance and expense.

Glucose monitoring is essential for type 1 patients who take insulin—and occasionally for certain type 2 patients prone to low blood sugar (hypoglycemia), particularly those on sulfonylurea drugs. But in general, type 2 diabetes can be managed effectively with the simple diet and exercise you'll discover in *The 30-Day Diabetes Cure*.

Two studies published in the *British Medical Journal* confirmed this. The first study split a group of newly diagnosed type 2 patients into equal groups: Those who self-monitored their blood sugar and those who didn't monitor at all. After 12 months, the diabetes (as measured by hemoglobin A1C testing, a method of measuring average blood sugar levels) was no better in the self-monitoring group.

The second study divided a separate population of type 2 patients into three groups: No monitoring, moderate monitoring, and intense monitoring. Not only did self-monitoring fail to improve diabetes control, it also cost more. More importantly, monitoring actually *decreased* the patients' quality of life because of frequent blood sugar testing and fretting.

Despite this well-published research, most doctors and the ADA continue to recommend self-monitoring. One has to wonder if the cost of test strips and glucose monitors has anything to do with this.

Diabetes Mistake #2: *"Lowering blood sugar with drugs is the most successful treatment for type 2 and prediabetes."*

In my experience, diabetes drugs are unnecessary for a majority of prediabetes and type 2 patients. The only instance in which I even consider drugs for these patients is in emergency situations, and even then I withdraw them as soon as possible. Not only are they unnecessary, but many of these drugs are dangerous—and have been proven so for years. With drugs, you can have ideal "numbers" and yet your diabetes will continue to progress relentlessly. In fact...

YOU CAN HAVE "PERFECT GLUCOSE" AND DIE FROM DIABETES

And that's exactly what a major study in 2008 called ACCORD proved.

For decades, doctors believed that if people with diabetes lowered their blood sugar to normal levels, they would negate their risk of dying from heart disease (the leading complication of diabetes). Incredibly, before ACCORD no research had ever studied this—it was just a strong held "belief."

ACCORD asked if maintaining normal blood sugar levels in people with type 2 diabetes would protect them from heart disease and lengthen their lives. (It also studied whether controlling cholesterol levels and blood pressure with drug therapy improved outcomes for diabetics. More about this part of ACCORD later.)

In the first part of the study, researchers divided 10,000 middle-aged and older people with type 2 diabetes into two groups. One group was told to aggressively maintain their hemoglobin

A1C at 6.0% (called "normal" by the American Diabetes Association) or lower. The other group took a more relaxed approach, allowing their blood sugar levels to hover between 7.0 and 7.9%.

The first group took glucose-lowering drugs and/or insulin shots (up to five or six per day) to reduce their blood sugar to this lower level. Some used insulin pumps. Some monitored their blood sugar seven to eight times a day.

The second group had an easier time of it, taking fewer drugs, lower doses and less frequent self-monitoring blood tests.

After four years, researchers made a shocking discovery: The patients lowering their blood sugar aggressively were suffering significantly more heart attacks and a higher rate of death compared to patients in the "relaxed" group. The problem was so serious that this part of the study was halted to protect the remaining participants.[1]

The medical community was stunned. The American Diabetes Association, which always pushed patients into lowering their blood sugar to these "normal" levels, was embarrassed. To this day, diabetes experts are still in a quandary about this.

In my experience, lowering blood sugar with drugs is the wrong approach. Not only does this give the person with diabetes a false sense of security—but these drugs have been shown to be dangerous. The safest, surest way to keep blood sugar levels at healthy levels is *not* to consume the foods and beverages that cause glucose and insulin to spike—and to reverse your cells' insulin resistance, which is the root of the problem. And this is incredibly simple to accomplish by simply following *The 30-Day Diabetes Cure* program.

Diabetes Mistake #3: *"Just take more insulin."* Taking drugs to make your pancreas produce more insulin—or injecting insulin itself—may make your doctor happy (because it brings your glucose levels down), but this is a short-sighted and potentially dangerous "Band-Aid" remedy.

A study reported in the March 2010 *New England Journal of Medicine* confirms this. Since doctors regard "postprandial hyperglycemia" (high blood sugar after eating) as dangerous, researchers proposed lowering it in patients who had prediabetes using a drug called *nateglinide*, which increases insulin secretion. The theory was that lowering postmeal blood sugar with more insulin would decrease the risk of heart disease.

But the results showed just the opposite effect. Not only did nateglinide *not* reduce the risk of developing full-blown diabetes, but it also failed to reduce the risk of heart disease or "cardiovascular events" (heart attacks). Further, it actually *increased* the risk of hypoglycemia (low blood sugar), a dangerous condition it its own right. There is another, institutional problem with blood sugar normalization: doctors' fears of having a patient die from hypoglycemia, for which they could be sued. So it's in the interest of physicians to keep their patients' blood sugars unnaturally

---

[1] Diabetes Study Partially Halted After Deaths by Gina Kolata; *New York Times*—February 7, 2008

16

high. If they die of heart attacks, as the ACCORD study indicates is more likely, they can say it was the "natural" consequence of the disease.

PROBLEMS CAUSED BY INCREASED INSULIN

Since insulin is the hormone that governs fat storage, high blood levels of it coupled with large amounts of dietary carbohydrate consumption encourage weight gain. (This can be a real conundrum if your doctor is nagging you to lose weight.)

More importantly, excess insulin in your bloodstream causes widespread inflammation, which is directly linked to metabolic syndrome, heart disease, Alzheimer's and cancer. For someone already at risk for heart disease (as all diabetics are), this combination increases the danger of premature death.

Another problem is that most diabetic complications—heart disease, peripheral neuropathy, vision loss, limb amputations, and others—are a direct result of high levels of blood glucose and insulin. Abnormally high levels of both (which is common with type 2 diabetes) damages blood vessels, causing them to become rigid or to leak.

Instead of simply supplying your cells with more insulin, they need to be "trained" to become more insulin-sensitive so they can better use your natural insulin—or reduce the amount you need to inject. This reduces your overall "insulin load." This is important because drugs that cause the pancreas to pump out more insulin actually *accelerate* the burning-out of beta cells, triggering type 1 (insulin-dependent) diabetes.

The 30-Day Diabetes Cure includes a number of safe, natural and easy ways to make your cells more sensitive to insulin. Even if you have type 1, you'll be able to reduce your insulin dose significantly. If you have type 2, you'll be preserving the life of the beta cells in your pancreas by not overworking them.

THE ONLY REAL SOLUTION

The easiest and best way to keep insulin and blood sugar levels normal is to eliminate fast-acting refined carbohydrates, such as starchy foods (bread, rice, pasta, etc.), and sugars from your diet—and to substitute slow-digesting carbs (vegetables and whole grains), while increasing the consumption of fiber-rich foods.

The ADA derides this low-carb approach, maintaining that diabetics are too lazy to adhere to it, although the strategy has worked fine for my patients. Had they followed the ADA diet, many of them would likely died years ago.

The low-carb strategy I'm advocating isn't the same as the Atkins Diet, although many people get the two confused. Whereas Atkins meals are high in animal protein with few carbohydrate foods (refined and complex), my approach minimizes refined carbs (hence, "low") while maximizing consumption of complex carbohydrate foods such as vegetables and whole grains.

The ADA maintains that low-carb diets should be avoided because there are no studies proving they are effective. That's not true. One study done in Sweden in 2006 found the diet to be very successful.

In the study, obese patients with type 2 diabetes followed a low-carbohydrate diet for 22 months. Most showed continuing improvements in blood sugar that were independent of weight loss. Medication use also was reduced. The average daily dosage of insulin among the insulin-dependent patients was cut in half.

"Many people are essentially cured of their [type 2] diabetes by low-carbohydrate diets, but that message is not getting out," says biochemistry professor Richard Feinman, PhD, of SUNY Downstate Medical Center, Brooklyn, NY.

While agreeing that carbohydrate restriction helps people with type 2 diabetes control their blood sugar, ADA spokesman Nathaniel G. Clark, MD, said that the ADA does not recommend very low-carb diets because "patients find them too restrictive."[2] But another explanation for ADA resistance could be the millions of dollars in revenue it receives by selling its Seal of Approval to food manufactures who market refined carbohydrate products. (See "Speaking of the ADA…" on page 22.)

Diabetes Mistake #4: *"Drugs protect against diabetic complications."* Sorry, but they don't. In recent research reported in the *New England Journal of Medicine (NEJM)*, the second part of the ACCORD study investigated whether using drug therapy to reduce high blood pressure and cholesterol in people with diabetes would reduce their risk of cardiovascular disease.

THE ANSWER WAS "NO"

Not only were these drugs ineffective—but they actually proved harmful.

Half of the 4,773 patients in the study took drugs to lower their systolic pressure (the top number) down to 120, which is considered normal. The other half had a goal of 140, which is higher than normal. Surprisingly (at least to the doctors who assumed it would), the lower blood pressure numbers *failed* to prevent heart attacks and cardiovascular deaths. And dangerous side effects from the drugs were plentiful, including the toxic load from taking up to three drugs just to lower blood pressure.

---

[2] http://diabetes.webmd.com/news/20060616/do-low-carb-diets-help-diabetes

The same issue of the *NEJM* reported on yet another failed study to lower blood pressure, this one involving 6,400 type 2 patients trying to lower their systolic blood pressure to 130. The result was a 50% *increase* in the risk of strokes, heart attacks and death.

Another aspect of the ACCORD study was equally fruitless. Lowering cholesterol to lower the risk heart attacks in people with diabetes is a common tactic cardiologists have tried. Prescribing cholesterol-lowering drugs called *statins* is the preferred conventional treatment, although these drugs have numerous adverse side effects and little-to-no evidence proving their ability to prevent heart attack or heart disease.

ACCORD researchers added a triglyceride-cholesterol drug called a *fibrate* to their patients' cocktail of pharmaceuticals, in concert with a statin drug. The results showed that combining the fibrate and a statin drug for diabetic patients did *not* produce any benefit in lower risk of cardiovascular disease or death as opposed to those taking only one or the other. [3]

A SAFER AND MORE EFFECTIVE APPROACH

Having healthy cholesterol levels and low blood pressure are certainly good for the health of your heart, but tinkering with blood pressure and cholesterol in a patient who already has dysfunctional blood sugar metabolism is not, in my view, the way to treat either the cardiovascular risk or the diabetes. Rather, I've found that once you the reverse the insulin resistance with proper diet and lifestyle modifications, cardiovascular risks–including high blood pressure and high triglycerides–resolve themselves. The drugs are unnecessary and counter-productive.

Doctors routinely see so many horrible diabetes complications that they've come to believe they're inevitable. To many, it's not a matter of "if" but *when*. That's why the official treatment for a newly diagnosed type 2 diabetic includes an ACE inhibitor (to control blood pressure and protect the kidneys), a cholesterol-lowering drug (to reduce the risk of heart attack, the leading cause of death in diabetes) and of course, medications that either control blood glucose or enhance insulin production (or both).

But these drugs are rarely effective and do absolutely *nothing* to reverse the underlying cause of diabetes: insulin resistance in your cells. Yet that's exactly where all the horrible complications of diabetes begin—and no amount of drugs or surgery will stop them. In truth, *no glucose-lowering drug has ever been shown to produce a reliable reduction in diabetic complications.* Neither has aggressive glucose monitoring.

Diabetics aren't dying because we don't know how to lower glucose—they're dying from complications. And they'll keep dying until we heal diabetes at the most fundamental level, using diet and increased physical activity.

---

[3] http://abcnews.go.com/Health/DiabetesNews/diabetes-intensive-cholesterol-blood-pressure-control-heart-risk/story?id=10098023

In the words of the Cleveland Clinic's Dr. Steve Nissen: "We've got to move beyond a glucose-centric approach. We have 10 classes of drugs to lower blood sugar…(but) we need ways to lower blood sugar that reduce the complications."[4]

Those sentiments are echoed by an overwhelmed family doctor in Logan County, West Virginia (which has the highest rate of diabetes in the entire US): "What happens is, we're throwing medicines at them, but medication is not a cure. We're not getting at the core of diabetes, which is diet and exercise. Some people are taking six, eight pills for their diabetes, checking their sugars four times a day. They just hate it." [5]

Diabetes Mistake #5: *"You've got to stop eating so much—and lose some weight."* The underlying message regarding type 2 and prediabetes is that they are self-inflicted diseases, just like smoking or AIDS. Conventional doctors say the reason you have diabetes is because you're overweight. But just the opposite is true: You're overweight because you have diabetes (or insulin resistance).

While there *is* a connection between losing weight and a reversal of diabetes, there's no definitive proof that this relationship is causal. There are many obese people who have zero symptoms of diabetes or insulin resistance. Plus, it's not unusual to find slender individuals with type 2. (I explain how this is possible in *The 30-Day Diabetes Cure*.)

IT'S ALL ABOUT LEPTIN

For many people, this scenario is caused by a deficiency in *leptin*, the "I'm full" hormone that tells your brain to stop eating and your pancreas to stop producing insulin. Scientists know that leptin resistance occurs years before insulin resistance and diabetes do. So, in my opinion, here's what your doctor *should* be telling you…

When your body doesn't produce enough leptin, you keep eating and your body holds on to weight, even if you're eating less. Being overweight, in turn, makes your body even more leptin-resistant, resulting in still more weight gain and more insulin production. Fortunately, following *The 30-Day Diabetes Cure* helps you break this cycle by increasing your body's leptin production with proper diet, physical activity, stress reduction, and a remarkable over-the-counter supplement that you'll read about in *The 30-Day Diabetes Cure* program.

THE PROBLEM WITH DIETING

The problem with weight-loss diets is that they usually have a beginning and an end. And in the middle, diets are a struggle to follow and stick with. (If you've ever been on one, you know how true this is.) That's why statistics show that they fail 95% of the time. Reason? Diets are no fun.

---

4 *Diabetes Rising* by Dan Hurley; Kaplan Publishing – p. 74
5 *Diabetes Rising* by Dan Hurley; Kaplan Publishing – p. 84

And the human nervous system is wired for pleasure and enjoyment. So if a diet plan doesn't taste good or feel good, the majority of people aren't going entertain it for very long.

The usual mindset is that pleasure and health can't possibly go together. We subconsciously believe that "pleasure" foods are bad for us and that healthful foods are boring. But as you'll see, this is completely mistaken. *The 30-Day Diabetes Cure* shows you how to eat for maximum health *and* pleasure. And you'll love every meal!

"WHICH WEIGHT-LOSS DIET SHOULD I GO ON, DOCTOR?"

Ask your physician this question and you'll probably be met with a shrug of the shoulders because most MDs just don't know the answer. Remember, a majority of doctors have virtually no training in nutrition.

"Just eat less and get some exercise," is the usual reply. (And you know how well that works.)

The 30-Day Diabetes Cure doesn't ask you to lose weight. Instead, you'll shed pounds naturally as you adopt a Diabetes Healing Lifestyle. As you may have guessed, the foods that cause diabetes are the same ones that pack on the pounds. So weight loss will be a natural, effortless by-product of reversing your diabetes.

You'll also learn a thoroughly enjoyable new approach to eating that fills your plate with delicious foods while keeping your blood sugar *naturally* low so your insulin doesn't rise. It may surprise you to learn that many of my patients have used this eating plan to get off their meds entirely (or reduce insulin injections if they're type 1). You'll read their inspiring success stories in *The 30-Day Diabetes Cure*.

I'LL NEVER ASK YOU TO DIET. *EVER.*

I'm not going to put you on some weird, boring weight-loss diet. And unlike most of the new, trendy "diabetes diets," my plan isn't vegetarianism in disguise. (Of course, you can choose to be a vegetarian on my eating plan if that suits you, but it's definitely not required.) With my patient-proven eating strategy, you'll never feel hungry—and you won't be embarrassed or tempted to cheat when you dine out with friends.

There are no fake-food meal replacement shakes or gimmicky energy bars involved. And if you've been plagued by constant carbohydrate cravings in the past, you'll discover a very simple way to reverse them so they'll be gone for good.

The 30-Day Diabetes Cure empowers you to make smart foods choices based on science—not somebody's opinion. You'll receive a thorough education about foods that heal diabetes, and about those that make it worse. *The 30-Day Diabetes Cure* is about healthful eating, not dieting.

And that's why it works so well: Because the weight comes off naturally. No weighing yourself. No counting carbs or calories. No more feeling guilty because you fell off your diet. Best of all, you're going to get that "lose-weight monkey" off your back for good.

Diabetes Mistake #6: *"Diet and lifestyle changes aren't that important."* Current diabetes drugs are approved by the FDA for use *along with* diet and exercise modifications. This means they're not approved for use in people who don't modify their diet and physical activity. But because doctors are focused on your blood sugar numbers, diet and exercise get forgotten. (Besides, insurance companies don't pay for education, remember?) This leads to Mistake #1, which gives patients permission to eat anything they want as long as they control their numbers with medications.

Instead of counseling and motivating you themselves, doctors usually refer diabetes patients to a Certified Diabetes Educator (CDE), who puts them on the officially sanctioned American Diabetes Association (ADA) diet. And this officially sanctioned diet is terrible for people with diabetes because it's essentially the same low-fat, high-carb diet that ignited the obesity epidemic in the 1980s. During that era, food manufacturers substituted extra sugars for the fats they removed, which actually *increased* the calorie content of these fat-free and low-fat food products!

As you learn more about *The 30-Day Diabetes Cure* program, you'll understand why people with diabetes actually *need* fats in their diet—as long as they're good fats. (*The 30-Day Diabetes Cure* will teach you the difference.)

SPEAKING OF THE ADA...

Much of the ADA's advice simply can't be trusted. Did you know the organization is largely supported by drug companies and food manufacturers? Its Seal of Approval essentially has been for sale since the ADA was founded. And it still is.

The ADA recently inked a new deal with Cadbury, the $1.2 million-a-year candy giant, whose products will now qualify for the ADA seal. Kraft Foods had a four-year, $1 million deal which allowed the ADA logo to appear on such products as SnackWell's cookies, Post Raisin Bran, Cream of Wheat cereal, and Sugar-Free Jell-O. (Could this be the real reason the ADA is against low-carb diets?) The *New York Times* reveals that it costs a minimum of $500,000 to even qualify for the ADA seal.

I find it scandalous that an organization with so much influence among doctors and consumers sells its "official medical approval" of food products that diabetics have no business eating. And who but giant corporations can afford this entry fee?

In another article published on November 25, 2006 ("In Diabetes Fight, Raising Cash and Keeping Trust"), the *Times* reports that the ADA received more than $23 million in support in a single year from the food and pharmaceutical industries. There's no mystery as to why. While the lion's share of the ADA's $210 million budget is spent promoting "treatments" (in other words, drugs), very little goes toward prevention, public awareness campaigns and patient education.

THE GLAXO CONNECTION

Right now, the estimated 41 million Americans currently classified as "prediabetic" (also called insulin-resistant) make up the most potentially lucrative sector of the diabetes market. These are people on the brink of developing type 2. Needless to say, this is a huge potential market and drug companies are scurrying to capture it.

One such pharmaceutical giant, GlaxoSmithKline, recently completed trials of a new drug to prevent prediabetes from turning into type 2. (This is reminiscent of the strategy that positioned cholesterol-lowering drugs called *statins* as being able to prevent heart disease.) The ADA is scheduled to publish its judgment on whether drug treatment for prediabetes in general—and perhaps Glaxo's new drug specifically—is warranted or recommended.

I'm not holding my breath in suspense for the answer and here's why: Glaxo donated $1 million to the ADA last year. In addition, all but one member of the ADA panel considering approval of the new Glaxo drug reported receiving direct payments or "research funding" from pharmaceutical companies on their financial disclosure forms, with three members receiving compensation from Glaxo.

THE ADA'S HISTORY WITH THE DRUG INDUSTRY

The ADA's relationship with Big Pharma dates back to 1940, when it was founded with a gift from the drug maker Eli Lilly. Twice in the past decade, the ADA's 12-member Executive Committee has been headed by former top executives of drug or medical equipment companies. The current ADA treasurer is the Director of Investor Relations for Johnson & Johnson. The ties to drug companies—and the drug industry in general—make it hard to believe the ADA is objective and impartial in its treatment choices.

Pharmaceutical companies sell $15 billion worth of diabetes drugs in the US each year, and the ADA is a lynchpin of their marketing strategy. The *New York Times* reports that companies continually advertise to doctors in ADA journals and announce new medicines at ADA conventions, where a coming-out party to tout a new drug can drive a stock price higher.

THERE *IS* ANOTHER WAY

The big business of diabetes is why I wrote *The 30-Day Diabetes Cure*. My plan empowers you to use education, the most potent medicine on earth, to help you improve and even reverse your diagnosis. Step-by-step and day-by-day, you'll read how to heal your diabetic or prediabetic condition…balance your blood sugar…stabilize and rebuild your insulin production…lose the weight that aggravates your condition, without dieting…strengthen your cardiovascular system…protect yourself from diabetic complications…and lengthen your life.

You can do this! In *The 30-Day Diabetes Cure,* you can read case studies of my patients who did it, too.

The Dangers of Diabetes Drugs

THE DANGERS OF DIABETES DRUGS

*"About 90% of the patients who visit doctors have conditions that
will either improve on their own or that are
out of reach of modern medicine's ability to solve."*

—NEW ENGLAND JOURNAL OF MEDICINE

THE "DIABETES BOOM" is in full swing. One way I can tell is by the number of invitations I receive from stockbrokers and mutual fund managers inviting me to cash in on the "enormous investment opportunity" in the global diabetes epidemic.

This sector of the financial industry is literally licking its chops at the potential wealth about to pour in. Did you notice how health care stocks skyrocketed at the very mention of "healthcare reform"? Investors know something we don't; and it's pretty obvious they assume they're going to make a fortune on this new legislation. And diabetes profits are high on the list.

It's heartbreaking to imagine the number of shiny new Mercedes, lavish vacation homes and CEO bonuses that will be generated from people's suffering. But it isn't surprising when you look at the history of the billions already made off various diseases.

Don't become one of the lives sacrificed to further enrich this corrupt system.

Chances are, if you have type 2 diabetes or prediabetes, your doctor is going to sell you hard on starting a drug regimen. He/she is going to make it sound "so easy" by telling you that going on a drug regimen will allow you to live a "normal" life. That you won't have to change your diet or lifestyle—and you'll still be able to eat whatever you want. Why do doctors push these drugs so aggressively?

BECAUSE THEY DON'T REALLY KNOW ANY OTHER WAY

Chances are, your physician may have seen one of the many studies proving beyond any doubt that simple diet and lifestyle modifications are the most effective way to prevent pre-diabetes from turning into type 2…to reverse type 2 if you already have it…and to lower the amount of insulin you have to take if you have type 1.

But this research is easy to ignore because these studies have no great champions to popularize them. On the other hand, drug companies send out armies of salespeople to tout their products at lavish "educational" conferences, lunches, weekend golf outings and with prime tickets to sporting events.

27

It's easy to see why studies showing the effectiveness of lifestyle modification get drowned out in the drug hoopla. As a result, most doctors haven't actually taken a close look at how safe and effective this approach really is. Most believe that a drug-free, diabetes-reversing program such as *The 30-Day Diabetes Cure* involves a restrictive, draconian diet coupled with slavish exercise—and that their patients just won't stick with it. *But in my experience, just the opposite is true.*

The 30-Day Diabetes Cure is an extremely easy plan to follow. The meals are delicious and you have a wide variety of foods from which to choose. And the physical activity is nothing more than simple walking, usually complimented by gentle yoga and stretching.

BUT WHERE'S THE MONEY IN THAT?

In 2009, the total cost of fighting diabetes and its complications in the US was $174 billion. Oral diabetes drugs accounted for around 39% of the total diabetes market. These are big bucks, indeed.

Metformin (Glucophage), the first-line therapy for type 2 diabetes—and now prediabetes—accounts for about 12% of these sales. Other glucose-lowering pills include *sulphonylureas*, *thiazolidinediones* (TZDs or glitazones), *glinides* and alpha-glucosidase inhibitors.

Excited financial forecasters are predicting the market for diabetes drugs, devices and monitoring systems will continue to grow at double-digit rates, reaching a value of over $55 billion by 2016. The market for insulin will expand over 18% next year alone, while continuous glucose monitoring systems will see growth of 48%. This translates into extraordinary profits for drug manufacturers and those who invest in them.

AND GUESS WHERE THESE PROFITS WILL COME FROM?

That's right: You. Even though you're still staggering from the mortgage meltdown…still paying for the massive bank bailout…still saddled with outrageous credit-card interest rates and hidden fees…still uncertain about your job security…and still challenged to make ends meet day-to-day—they're planning to squeeze the last red cent out of you with fear tactics and lies about diabetes. But I'm not going to let them get away with it. And I hope you won't either. As the saying goes…

"IF YOU'RE NOT OUTRAGED, YOU'RE NOT PAYING ATTENTION"

Scandal after scandal is awakening more Americans to the reality of just how few freedoms we have left. Many of us are beginning to realize that we're being lied to by politicians who wrap themselves in the flag of patriotism when they want us to vote a certain way, but who are secretly influenced by lobbyists and corporations seeking legislation that benefits them (and only them). Example: Fast food and soda lobbyists spent more than $57,000,000 in 2009 to sway our elected representatives in squashing the harm these industries inflict on the public's health. Go to *http://www.opensecrets.org/lobby/indusclient.php?year=2009&iname=N01&id=food&beverage* to see how much each company actually spent. You'll be shocked. It's no exaggeration to say that diabetes may be the world's first corporate sponsored disease.

If this makes you angry, it should. Today, corporations dominate our government. Laws are written that overwhelmingly favor industries at the expense of private citizens. Meanwhile, taxpayers foot the bill for billion-dollar bailouts to banks. Consumers suffer under oppressive credit card rates, unfair mortgage practices, rising unemployment, out-of-control health insurance premiums and monopolistic control of life's essential resources and services.

AND THE MEDICAL INDUSTRY IS NO EXCEPTION

Did you know that doctors are largely educated by drug company reps—especially about new drugs? These days, virtually all of the studies "proving" the value of pharmaceutical drugs are created and run by the companies who make them. If this sounds like the fox guarding the henhouse, you're right.

Drug companies have more influence over US doctors, medical school curriculum and today's treatments protocols than you might realize. I'm betting you didn't know that…

- Drug companies spend $16 billion annually to directly influence doctors. That's $10,000 for every single physician in the US.

- A national survey reveals that virtually *all* doctors have some type of financial relationship with the pharmaceutical industry.

- More than 80% of Americans think drug companies have too much influence over the Food and Drug Administration.[1]

- Greater than half the residency programs that train US physicians accept financial support from the drug industry, paying for young doctors' meals, housing, textbooks and education.[2]

Dr. Jerome Kassirer, former editor at the *New England Journal of Medicine*, summarized the problem perfectly when he said: "[Financial ties] are dangerous when doctors are so beholden to the company that they withhold safety concerns or push the newest or most expensive products when they aren't necessarily best for the patient." This is exactly what's happening, folks.

Drug companies have a long history of "cooking the books" on their studies, often withholding data on adverse side effects (as in the heart attacks and strokes caused by the arthritis

---

[1] Consumer Reports National Research Center
[2] Doctor Training Aided by Drug Industry Cash; *The New York Times*—February 23, 2010

drug Vioxx) or exaggerating a drug's benefits (like the makers of cholesterol-lowering statins do). And this is especially true for diabetes drugs. Let me give you just a few examples...

THE ORINASE ODYSSEY

In 1957, the Upjohn Company introduced a sugar-lowering sulfa drug (the technical name is *sulfonylurea*) called Orinase (Tolbutamide) that forever transformed diabetes treatment, including how the disease is defined.

Orinase was promoted to the medical community as a new wonder drug that could halt diabetes and also prevent its progression in *symptomless patients* who had a mild, usually undiagnosed form of the disease—what we now refer to as prediabetes.

Upjohn was in fact creating a new disease category ("hidden diabetes") which would greatly expand its potential market, even though the company provided no clinical evidence. Everyone simply assumed that lowering blood sugar levels would also lower the risks of diabetic complications. Upjohn even hinted that Orinase might even prevent this mild form of diabetes from becoming more severe.

By the end of the 1960s, more than 800,000 US patients were taking Orinase every day for mild, non-symptomatic diabetes, based on the assumption that the pill reduced their long-term risk for developing type 2 and diabetic complications including heart disease. But a bombshell dropped on May 20, 1970.

THIS DRUG WAS KILLING PATIENTS

When the results were released from the largest diabetes study ever conducted to track mortality (death) rates of diabetics who were on pills, on insulin or using diet modifications alone, the findings were stunning. Independent researchers found that 12.7% of diabetics taking Orinase had died of heart disease, compared with less than 5% who were given a placebo (a pill containing no medicine). This means the drug was causing more than *twice* the heart disease deaths compared with *doing absolutely nothing*. By contrast, the death rate of patients taking insulin was the same as for those who were managing their condition with diet alone.

Three weeks later, the FDA sent a letter to physicians recommending that sulfonylurea drugs should no longer be prescribed because of the harm they were doing. Strangely, *the ADA rejected the FDA's response, claiming it saw no need to abandon the use of these drugs.*

Despite the FDA's advice, physicians continued to prescribe Orinase and other sulfonylurea drugs. By 1975, some 1.5 million people were taking them, even though the National Institutes of Health (NIH) estimated they were causing 15,000 deaths annually. The FDA's weak response? Manufacturers were required to issue warning labels alerting patients to the dangers.

Curiously, the warning label wasn't put in place until 1984—9 years later!—and it still remains on all sulfonylureas, including a second generation of drugs that are far more powerful than Orinase. It's estimated that since the time of its introduction, Orinase and other sulfonylureas have been responsible for "tens of thousands of deaths." Upjohn (now a casualty of corporate mergers) stopped making Orinase in 2000, though a generic form is still being marketed and prescribed.

NEW DRUGS, NEW DANGERS

In the 1990s, a new class of sugar-lowering drugs made its appearance. Metformin, a drug similar to *phenformin* (banned in 1977 due to potentially fatal side effects) debuted in 1994. Doctors favored metformin because it didn't trigger dangerously low blood-sugar levels and seemed to cause weight loss in patients, instead of weight gain.

Marketed under the brand name Glucophage, it since has become the best-selling pill for type 2 and prediabetes. Many physicians consider it to be the safest and most effective medication for newly diagnosed patients.

But when tested head-to-head against nondrug lifestyle modifications over a three-year period in the nationwide Diabetes Prevention Program (DPP), metformin did only *half* as well at controlling blood sugar levels compared to lifestyle modifications.[3] This is an extremely important point to note. Even though diet and lifestyle modifications are proven to be *twice* as effective as the best-selling glucose-lowering medication, doctors still rely on the drug as their primary treatment protocol. One has to wonder why. Obviously, something other than clinically based evidence is behind this. But on with the story…

REZULIN—THE LIVER KILLER

Rezulin, created by Warner-Lambert, was touted as the next superstar diabetes drug. Because it targeted insulin resistance in the muscles, it was supposed to help patients use less insulin to normalize blood glucose levels. The FDA fast-tracked its approval in January 1997 (again, one wonders why, given the dangerous nature of previous diabetes drugs)—and sure enough, serious problems began to surface just *months* after its introduction.

Dozens of Rezulin patients were hospitalized with liver problems, some of them fatal. Rezulin's apparent liver toxicity prompted Britain to ban it, but the FDA decided that a warning to US physicians was sufficient. It wasn't. By March of 1999, the number of liver failure cases among US patients reached 43—with 28 of them dying. A high-ranking FDA official called Rezulin one of the most dangerous drugs in America, but the agency continued to defend it. Rezulin wasn't

[3] Diabetes Prevention Program Research Group

banned until March 2000, after being implicated in 391 deaths. During that time it brought in more than $2 billion in sales for Warner-Lambert.

THE DEADLY DIABETES DRUG STILL ON THE MARKET

By 2007, US physicians had more than 18 different glucose-lowering medications from which to choose, including Avandia from GlaxoSmithKline. This was another drug fast-tracked just like Rezulin. Yet none of these new drugs had *ever* been proven conclusively to be effective or safe, especially when compared to simple diet and lifestyle modification. And no study ever confirmed that any of these drugs protected patients against the most fatal complication of diabetes: Heart disease, the cause of death in 75% of people with diabetes.

In fact, a prominent study published in the *New England Journal of Medicine* showed just the opposite: Avandia actually increased the risk of heart attack by 43%—and cardiovascular fatalities by a whopping 64%—compared to patients not on the drug. That meant that *not taking* Avandia actually doubled a type 2 patient's chances of avoiding a cardiovascular event. (An Alice in Wonderland moment if I've ever seen one.)

THE DRUG-MAKER HID THE DANGERS FROM THE PUBLIC

Senate investigations underway in early 2010 show that as far back as 2003, Glaxo's own studies revealed that Avandia caused an alarming number of heart problems, but that the company hid this from the public and the FDA.[4]

Even though Avandia may have been responsible for as many as 83,000 heart attacks, Glaxo continued to aggressively market it, persuading doctors to recommend the drug—and actually threatening doctors who publicly suggested that Avandia was dangerous.[5]

"We've been warning about this for two and a half years," says Steven Nissen, MD, a prominent cardiologist at the Cleveland Clinic who ran the Avandia study. "There really isn't a good reason for physicians to continue to prescribe the drug. It's time to get it off the market."[6]

Of course, Glaxo didn't agree—and with good reason: Before these revelations, Avandia was the world's best-selling diabetes drug, with more than $3 billion in sales 2006 alone.

If you're currently taking Avandia, I urge you to immediately discuss with your doctor switching to a less risky drug. A newly-released study shows that if every diabetic now taking Avandia was switched to Actos (a similar, but safer drug), about 500 heart attacks and 300 cases of heart failure would be averted *each and every month*.

---

[4] Diabetes Drug Harms Heart, U.S. Concludes; *The New York Times* (Front Page)—February 20, 2010
[5] Diabetes Drug Harms Heart, U.S. Concludes; *The New York Times* (Front Page)—February 20, 2010
[6] *Diabetes Rising* by Dan Hurley; Kaplan Publishing—p. 74

WHAT IF YOU ACTUALLY *NEED* A DIABETES DRUG?

Glucose-lowering medications may have a role to play in the short-term, but all they can achieve is keeping your blood sugar within a specific range. This won't cure diabetes—because it isn't simply a disease of high blood sugar. Rather, it's a metabolic disorder that affects every organ and hormonal system in your body. Simply lowering your glucose levels with a drug (or drugs) is like furiously mopping up water from a broken pipe, instead of repairing the leak.

These drugs also contain serious risks. For instance, glucose-lowering medications increase the risk of hypoglycemic (low blood sugar) episodes because they cause blood sugar to drop too quickly. This can be extremely dangerous.

Glucose medications also do nothing to help protect, repair or regenerate your beta cells, the cells in your pancreas that manufacture insulin. But some studies show that certain supplements, vitamins and foods may achieve exactly that—which is why we're so convinced this is best way to treat your condition. (See *How to Heal Your Pancreas*, page 56.)

In the end, you *may* actually need a drug, depending on your individual situation. But I urge you not to give in until you go all out with the diet and lifestyle approach described in *The 30-Day Diabetes Cure*.

Just be sure to do this in partnership with your physician or healthcare provider. It's extremely important you tackle this as a team—and your doctor's enthusiastic participation is essential. If he/she won't provide it, maybe it's time to look for a different doctor. The medical community is waking up to the value on non-drug approaches (albeit slowly) and there are plenty of open-minded practitioners who are willing to support you in trying these strategies first. It's up to you to find one.

YOU *CAN* ESCAPE THIS DRUG MERRY-GO-ROUND

Another drawback of drugs is that once you start medications, it's very hard to get your doctor to discontinue them. These days, most physicians tend to prescribe multiple medications for diabetes: A drug (or drugs) to lower blood sugar…a cholesterol-lowering drug to "protect" against heart disease…an ACE inhibitor to protect the kidneys…and also anti-hypertensive medication to control blood pressure. Each of these drugs has its own list of side effects, which may require still more drugs to alleviate. Are you getting dizzy from this endless pharmaceutical merry-go-round? I urge you to hop off while you still can. The 30-Day Diabetes Cure will show you how.

Ultimately, it's your responsibility to you to educate yourself and be aware of the numerous mistakes doctors are currently making in the treatment of all types of diabetes. I urge you to read *Mistakes Doctors Are Making with Diabetes* (page 13) to focus your attention on these dangerous treatment errors so you can avoid them. The last thing you want is to become another medical mistake.

Dodging Diabetes Complications

DODGING DIABETES COMPLICATIONS

"Life is not merely to be alive, but to be well."

—MARCUS VALERIUS MARTIAL

DIABETES COMPLICATIONS are devastating. Once they begin developing, it's difficult to turn them around. It's far wiser, easier, and cheaper to prevent and reverse the underlying condition that leads to them. And that's what this Special Report is all about.

The first step on this path is to choose the lifestyle modifications I describe in *The 30-Day Diabetes Cure* so you can get off glucose-lowering medications, because your body will never heal as long as you're on them. Let's examine step-by-step the health problems that diabetes poses—and how you can dodge these deadly complications.

THE DREADFUL COMPLICATIONS OF DIABETES

The tragic complications of diabetes can be seen everywhere you look—from the sightless stranger to the legless woman in a wheelchair. A generation ago we would have assumed "war veteran." Today a far safer assumption is "veteran of the war with diabetes."

Other victims include the 60-year-old who's afraid to lift his grandson because grandpa's feet and fingers are nearly numb from neuropathy and in agony from frequent debilitating pain. Or the stressed-out husband carrying a 40-pound belly, angry and frustrated because he's lost his sex drive to diabetes. Then there's the woman with Alzheimer's who can't recognize the face of her daughter. And the young girl on the playground, too obese to be active. Every one of them is a ticking time bomb.

TICK, TICK, TICK...

Diabetes begins in your endocrine (hormone) system. Once hormones go awry, the entire body is at risk for massive malfunction, with a broad range of crushing complications affecting everything from the circulatory system, kidneys, liver, eyes, muscles, heart and brain. Even with early diagnosis, diabetes steals the eyesight of 24,000 Americans every year;[1] 250,000 suffer kidney failure;[2] and 90,000 have limbs amputated.[3]

---

[1] http://forecast.diabetes.org/magazine/your-ada/time-every-purpose
[2] http://www.nkdep.nih.gov/news/releases/world-diabetes-day-focuses-on-preventing-diabetic-kidney-disease.htm
[3] http://findarticles.com/p/articles/mi_m0PDG/is_6_4/ai_n15882202/

People with diabetes are overwhelmingly at risk for heart disease, with some form of heart dysfunction being the cause of death in 75% of diabetic fatalities. The average life span of a diabetic is 15 to 20 years shorter—and risk of death is 400% greater—compared with someone without the disease.

Forgive me for being graphic, but diabetes complications are horrifically destructive. Vital organs fail, while digits and limbs must be removed one by one. According to the CDC, diabetes is the leading cause of kidney failure and dialysis, plus blindness and foot or leg amputations among adults.

THE HIGH COST OF DIABETES

Then there are extra medical expenses diabetes patients must pay year after year; an inevitable drain on personal finances and a major cause of bankruptcies and foreclosures today. These include costs for hospital care, dialysis treatments, the never-ending cocktail of pharmaceuticals, frequent doctor visits and diabetes supplies, including test strips, insulin pumps and neuropathy stockings. These add up to thousands of dollars per patient per year, all to "manage" an illness that continues to progress despite the enormous efforts to merely slow it down.

But this burdensome price tag pales compared to the misery and suffering the advancing diabetic must endure. Unfortunately, many people continue to believe that if they gobble a handful of pills or inject more insulin, they'll be fine. This simply isn't true. Diabetes continues to progress unless you step in, take charge of your life and turn the underlying cause of this terrible disease around.

CURRENT DRUG TREATMENT IS POWERLESS AGAINST COMPLICATIONS

Doctors routinely see so many horrible diabetes complications that they've come to believe they're inevitable. To many, it's not a matter of "if" but when. That's why current treatment for a newly diagnosed type 2 patient includes an ACE inhibitor (to control blood pressure and protect the kidneys), a cholesterol-lowering drug (to reduce the risk of heart attack, the leading cause of death in diabetes) and of course, medications that either control blood glucose or enhance insulin production (or both).

But these drugs are rarely effective and do absolutely nothing to reverse the underlying cause of diabetes: insulin resistance in your cells. Yet that's exactly where all the horrible complications of diabetes begin—and no amount of drugs or surgery will stop them. In truth, no glucose-lowering drug has ever been shown to produce a reliable reduction in diabetic complications. Neither has aggressive glucose monitoring.

People with diabetes aren't dying because we don't know how to lower glucose—they're dying from complications. And they'll keep dying until we heal diabetes at the most fundamental level, using diet and increased physical activity.

NEW STUDY PROVES THESE DRUGS ARE DANGEROUS

Recently released research proves that these drugs are not only worthless in fighting diabetes, but actually harmful. The *New England Journal of Medicine* (NEJM) reported in March 2010 on the ACCORD study which theorized that lowering the high blood pressure of people with diabetes would reduce the risk of cardiovascular disease.

■ Half of the 4,773 patients in the study took drugs to lower their systolic pressure (the top number) down to 120, which is considered normal. The other half had a goal of 140, which is higher than normal. Surprisingly (at least to the doctors who assumed it would), the lower blood pressure numbers failed to prevent heart attacks and cardiovascular deaths. And dangerous side effects from the drugs were plentiful, including the toxic load from taking up to three drugs just to lower blood pressure.

■ The same issue of the NEJM reported on yet another failed study to lower blood pressure, this one involving 6,400 type 2 patients trying to lower their systolic blood pressure to 130. The result was a 50% increase in the risk of strokes, heart attacks and death.

■ Another aspect of the ACCORD study confirms that the medical current obsession with drugs and numbers does nothing to save diabetics from heart attacks. Lowering cholesterol is a common tactic cardiologists have tried—and failed with. Prescribing cholesterol-lowering drugs called statins is the preferred conventional treatment, although these drugs have numerous adverse side effects and little-to-no evidence proving their ability to prevent heart attack or heart disease.

■ In this most recent study, doctors wanted to add a triglyceride-cholesterol drug called a *fibrate* to their patients' cocktail of pharmaceuticals, in concert with a statin drug. The results showed that combining the fibrate and a statin drug for diabetic patients did not produce any benefit in lower risk of cardiovascular disease or death as opposed to those taking only one or the other.

Having healthy cholesterol levels and low blood pressure are certainly good for the health of your heart, but tinkering with blood pressure and cholesterol in a patient who already has dysfunctional blood sugar metabolism is not, in my view, the way to treat either the cardiovascular risk or the diabetes. Rather, I've found that once you the reverse the insulin resistance with proper diet and lifestyle modifications, cardiovascular risks—including high blood pressure and high triglycerides—resolve themselves. The drugs are unnecessary and counterproductive.

Advanced diabetes is particularly grim. Even with all those drugs, all that monitoring and all those insulin injections, there's the emotional trauma that accompanies going blind, losing your fingertips, or having a limb amputated. Even in its early stages, people with diabetes have a higher incidence of depression than the general population. And the care-giving burden borne by family members is draining, with later-stage diabetic life revolving around constant drugs, dialysis treatments, doctor visits and late night trips to the emergency room.

THE POWER OF LIFESTYLE CHANGES

Here's the confounding irony: Reversing the root causes of diabetes itself costs virtually nothing when you follow *The 30-Day Diabetes Cure*. That's not just my opinion and clinical experience…

This has been confirmed by Centers for Disease Control and Prevention (CDC). Its Diabetes Prevention Program (DPP) studied more than 3,200 adults on the brink of developing type 2 diabetes. They compared the effectiveness of "Lifestyle Intervention Strategies" (healthy diet and moderate physical activity) with "Pharmacological Agent," in this case the commonly prescribed *metformin* (Glucophage). It is the first major clinical trial of Americans at high risk for type 2 diabetes confirming that lifestyle changes prevent or delay the disease significantly.[4]

■ Lifestyle changes reduced participants' risk of getting type 2 diabetes by 58%, while metformin reduced their risk by 31%. This means lifestyle adjustments are twice as effective.

■ Lifestyle modifications were equally effective for all ages and all ethnic groups.

Within the three-year period, lifestyle modifications cost $16,000 per case of diabetes prevented, while metformin cost $31,000 per case of diabetes prevented. *That's twice the expense.*

The conclusion to be drawn from this definitive research is that whether you have diabetes or prediabetes, if you take over your own lifestyle "intervention" with the help of my 30-day plan, you can be living proof of the clear-cut results in your blood sugar, blood pressure, cholesterol, triglycerides and thickening blood.

More than $400 billion is spent each year to combat diabetes globally, but less than one percent of that sum funds education, now the most successful and effective treatment. But that's just part of the diabetes story.

SOME VERY SCARY NUMBERS

Consider these stark realities:

■ Every 10 seconds two people develop diabetes and one dies from diabetes-related complications.

---

[4] CDC Statement On Results Of Diabetes Prevention program http://www.cdc.gov/diabetes/news/docs/dpp.htm

- One in 12 Americans currently has diabetes or prediabetes—with as many as one in every three born after 2000 at risk for diabetes in the future.

- The diabetes rate is two to four times higher for African-Americans, Hispanic/Latino Americans, American Indians and Asians.

- Heart disease accounts for 75% of diabetes-related deaths in individuals 65 and older.

- 75% of people with diabetes have significant problems with high cholesterol, high blood pressure and hypercoagulation (excessive blood clotting), a leading cause of stroke and heart attack.

- Diabetes causes a whopping 44% of new kidney failure cases.

- Up to 70% of people with diabetes have some level of central nervous system damage. This is neuropathy, causing tingling and relentless pain in the hands and feet that can eventually lead to amputation.

- Serious pregnancy complications occur in pregnant women whose diabetes is not well controlled.

And yet diabetes isn't an infectious disease. It's a lifestyle condition that can be avoided… and reversed once patients are properly educated on how to defeat it, on how to avoid drugs that merely suppress symptoms…and save themselves from its horrible complications.

REDUCING YOUR RISK

Numerous studies prove that maintaining near-normal blood glucose significantly decreases chronic diabetes complications—although glucose-lowering drugs are an ineffective (if not impossible) way to achieve this. Take a look at these citations, but please keep reading for my take on them…

- Improved glycemic control contributes to significant risk reduction to the eyes, kidneys and nervous system, according to two landmark studies. The Diabetes Control and Complications Trial (DCCT), involving patients with type 1 diabetes, showed a 63% relative risk reduction in retinopathy, 54% reduction in kidney damage and 60% risk in neuropathy.

- Up to 21% risk reduction in retinopathy and 33% risk reduction in kidney damage in type 2 diabetics was reported by the UK Prospective Diabetes Study (UKPDS). A smaller study of patients with type 2, done in Japan, showed risk reductions of 69% for retinopathy and 70% for kidney disease in those who achieved tighter glycemic control, compared to the control group.

Understand that the medical industry has responded to studies like these with a drug cornucopia that's supposed to tightly manage blood sugar, cholesterol and blood pressure. All this to achieve your specific, almost "magical" numeric objectives.

An enormous problem, which doctors rarely mention, is that all these drugs come with life-threatening hazards of their own. Pharmaceuticals may reduce some risk, but without re-shaping your fundamental way of living, the disease inevitably continues to progress, as do its complications.

Solid research proves beyond a doubt that you can heal your diabetes safely, naturally and *without* resorting to impossible fad diets and medieval surgical interventions. The handfuls of damaging drugs that target your symptoms do nothing for your underlying condition. *The 30-Day Diabetes Cure* shows you how to stop diabetes in its tracks. In the meantime it's important to know what's going on inside your body.

GET TESTED

Regardless of where you currently live on the diabetes spectrum—pre-diabetes, type 1 or type 2—you need these tests regularly while you're following *The 30-Day Diabetes Cure*. They'll not only keep you and your doctor in close touch with your improvements, but also provide concrete results as you start using my natural approach.

I urge you to regularly record your results for these tests. As they improve, you'll want them for bragging about, but they're also invaluable as you work with your doctor to make decisions on altering your medications over time. Some of these tests are routine, others are not as well known by general practitioners. Here are my recommendations:[5]

Fasting Blood Sugar and Glucose Tolerance

A fasting blood sugar test is performed at your doctor's office, usually in the morning after you've fasted for ten to 12 hours. A glucose tolerance test evaluates the amount of sugar in your blood after an eight-hour fast and two hours after you swallow a very sweet liquid.

Why you need these tests. They measure the amount of glucose in your blood and help diagnose prediabetes and diabetes. Fasting sugar levels of 100-125mg/dL (milligrams per deciliter) indicate prediabetes, as does glucose tolerance test results between 140 and 199 mg/dL. Both signal a risk of developing diabetes.

When to take them. Work with your doctor to determine the best test schedule, especially if you're controlling your blood sugar naturally on *The 30-Day Diabetes Cure*. Why? Because most people following my plan require less supplemental medication. Continuing your usual dose can

---

[5] http://www.labtestsonline.org/

actually put you in a low blood sugar situation (hypoglycemia). Getting off your meds entirely is certainly the goal, but be sure to keep your doctor informed while you're actively making changes, so he/she can make the appropriate adjustments to your test schedule and medications.

Serum (Blood) Insulin

This isn't a routine test; you must request it. If you have chronically-high insulin, you're likely a prediabetic and heading for serious complications. High insulin levels put you on the road to diabetes—even if your blood sugar is within the normal range. In fact, excess insulin circulating in your blood means your pancreas is already working overtime pumping out insulin to "unlock" cells and usher in glucose for energy. But high blood levels of insulin also indicate your cells are becoming resistant to insulin's "knock on the door," and may even be in the process of "changing the locks" so insulin won't be able to get in at all in the future.

If you have consistent, slightly high blood sugar over time—even if your readings are in the normal range—your pancreas will be adversely affected. Remember, this is the first evidence you're entering the danger zone. Your cells are already becoming resistant to insulin's knock at the door.

In short, elevated insulin indicates the beta-cells in your pancreas are already overtaxed. Long before you suffer the consequences of formal insulin resistance, your blood knows—and shows—what's coming.

Why you need this test. Having this test regularly serves as an advance warning of complications to come. High insulin levels should prompt you to immediately start *The 30-Day Diabetes Cure*, which will dramatically reduce your insulin, reverse the dysfunction and very possibly repair damage already done to your organs, arteries and nerves. Plus, if you have chronically high insulin, you're being exposed to inflammatory chemicals and high levels of *cortisol*, an extremely damaging stress hormone that can raise your chances for cancer in addition to diabetes.

When to take it. Get this test every time you have your blood glucose levels tested, or least once a year. Serum insulin results are best viewed in relation to your fasting blood sugar glucose reading. Compared to each other, the ratio of glucose to insulin is ideally greater than 10 to 1.

Healthy insulin levels themselves are between 5 and 10 microunits/milliliter (ml). Once you exceed 10 microunits, your risk of developing diabetes grows. Over 25, you're in real trouble. It goes without saying that I'd prefer you start *The 30-Day Diabetes Cure* before you ever get close to 25.

If you've had type 2 diabetes for a few years, you and your doctor should be aware that your pancreas is wearing out and may not be releasing much insulin. This can result in a low serum insulin reading—but not in a good way. Rather, it can signal that you're close to becoming insulin-dependent.

Hemoglobin A1C (HBA1C)

This is a standard lab test used to screen for prediabetes and monitor those who already have it. Because the A1C reveals your blood sugar *average* over a three-month period with a single test, it's one of the best ways to understand the fluctuations in your blood sugar over time. Even though it is currently the best test for diagnosing diabetes, it can still miss people who are developing prediabetes, so be sure you receive the blood glucose and serum insulin tests as well.

Why you need this test. The A1C evaluates how much glycated hemoglobin A1C is circulating in your blood. What exactly does this mean? Hemoglobin is the aspect of your red blood cells that delivers oxygen to all the cells in your body, 90% of which is termed hemoglobin A (as is A1C). When blood sugar is excessive, glucose molecules hijack the red blood cell and occupy oxygen's usual position, turning it into "glycated" hemoglobin.

Because the normal life span of a red blood cell is about 120 days, glycated hemoglobin cells die and are replaced with new (non-glycated) red blood cells during this time period. The A1C test shows the average glycated hemoglobin level over a three month period, reflecting the ups and downs of your blood sugar. The usual glucose blood test is more like an "at this moment" snapshot of your blood sugar, while the A1C is like a video. This "movie" is a more accurate, wide-frame look at your metabolism.

- In 2009, British scientists reported in the medical journal *Lancet* that diabetics who drive down their A1C by just one percent over five years can lower their heart attack risk by 17%.

- A 10-year study by the National Institute of Diabetes and Digestive and Kidney Diseases found that people who control their A1C succeeded in lowering their risk for eye disease by 76%, for kidney disease by 50% and for nerve disease (which leads to amputation) by 60%.

How do you lower A1C? The most effective way is by changing your diet to eliminate processed, refined carbohydrates and sugary drinks, while building your diet around fresh whole foods such as fruits and vegetables, naturally-raised meats and dairy products, and beneficial monounsaturated fats like those found in nuts and olive oil. Regular physical activity also helps accelerate reductions in A1C. This is the basis of *The 30-Day Diabetes Cure* plan.

When to take it. You should have an A1C test two to four times a year, or as often as your doctor recommends. Fasting is not required. A1C results are presented as a percentage, with normal A1C between 4% and 6%. People with diabetes should aim for scores around 7%.

More aggressive reductions (6% or lower), once the goal of medical intervention, recently has been shown not to be any more affective, and may actually increase the risk of complications.

Thyroid Tests[6]

A poorly functioning thyroid can undermine that blood sugar control. Underactive thyroid (hypothyroidism) is common in people with type 2 diabetes; plus nearly one-third of women with type 1 have some kind of thyroid disorder, often overactive (hyperthyroid). Because the symptoms and signs of diabetes and thyroid disorders are similar, thyroid problems are easily overlooked by doctors.

In addition, even when the standard TSH test, which shows how much *thyroid-stimulating hormone* (TSH) is being produced, reveals a "normal" thyroid, you can still be living with the symptoms of low thyroid.

Also ask to be tested for Reverse T3 (rT3) thyroid hormone. Reverse T3 blocks the action of active thyroid, so it actually works against you. If your rT3 is high—even if your TSH numbers are in the normal range—you can still have a low-functioning thyroid.

Your rT3, the "inactivity hormone" goes up in the presence of damaging inflammation. This is the hormone that says, "Slow down. Take a nap. Don't do anything even mildly strenuous. Why not just sleep for a week?" When it's high, you're the opposite of energetic.

Your body relies on the thyroid gland to keep your overall metabolism clipping along—also for burning fat for fuel. With low thyroid-function, you not only have no energy, but your body holds on to body fat. In addition to dragging around, you also gain weight. Normal levels of thyroid hormone, on the other hand, protect you from diabetes because they improve insulin levels so your energy system stays in balance. Without enough thyroid hormone, insulin resistance, high insulin levels and weight gain occur.

Why you need these tests. Because of its connection to diabetes, it's as essential to track your thyroid levels as it is your blood sugar and insulin. Having low levels of thyroid hormone can cause insulin resistance and lead to weight gain, which prompts even higher insulin levels and more belly fat.

Low thyroid function decreases your insulin needs, while high thyroid can snarl glucose control. Correcting for low thyroid produces quick elevated energy levels, weight loss and improved insulin sensitivity—and eventually, better blood glucose control.

When to take them. If you feel sluggish and tired, or if you're gaining weight even though you're eating habits haven't changed, ask your doctor to check your TSH and your rT3.

Urinalysis

This is an inexpensive and effective way to check for diabetes. If you have excess glucose circulating in your bloodstream, your kidneys become overloaded and can't filter it all, thus

---

[6] Thyroid Disease and Diabetes http://www.thyroidtoday.com/PatientResources1.asp

dumping the extra into your urine. Urinalysis also checks your levels of *microalbumin*, a protein that moves into urine via the kidneys in the same way as excess sugar.

Why you need this test. Excess glucose in your urine is a clear indicator that you have too much in your bloodstream. Microalbumin in your urine signals that your kidneys aren't filtering well and may already be compromised. (Kidney disease is a common complication of diabetes.)

When to take it. Your doctor should check your urine at every visit.

Cholesterol and Triglycerides

Doctors call these lipids, (meaning fats). Checking their levels is just as important as monitoring blood sugar and blood pressure so you can avoid diabetes complications.

Why you need these tests. They check your level of three different fats: HDL cholesterol, a beneficial lipoprotein that cleans out LDL from your arteries and veins; LDL, a troublesome lipoprotein linked to heart risk; and triglycerides, fats which are converted by insulin and stored in fat cells. Elevated LDL and triglycerides can indicate artery hardening and other cardiovascular risks.

When to take them. Once a year for most people, unless you've been diagnosed with heart disease and/or diabetes. Aim for these target numbers…

- LDL, 100 mg/dl or less

- HDL, over 40 mg/dl for men and over 50 mg/dl for women

- Triglycerides, less than 150 mg/dL

BLOOD SUGAR SELF-MONITORING: MY APPROACH MAY SURPRISE YOU

Most people with diabetes monitor their own blood sugar one or more times daily by pricking their skin and putting a drop of blood on a glucose strip. The strip is then read by a glucose meter, which reports your sugar level. Type 1 diabetics monitor their glucose so they can adjust their insulin dose accordingly; and patients following *The 30-Day Diabetes Cure* are often able to dramatically lower their doses.

I don't encourage my type 2 patients to perform daily glucose monitoring except in special cases. This is quite different from the current medical approach. But I recommend it because I strongly believe we need to move away from the mentality that good food choices are a penalty for bad numbers. In other words, when sugar goes up, most type 2's feel they need to "watch" their diet more closely. Add when their numbers come back down, they are more likely to reward themselves by "cheating."

I view this in precisely the opposite way. If you're like my patients who use glucose monitoring as positive reinforcement ("I can actually see I'm doing better on Dr. Ripich's plan"), I don't see anything wrong with monitoring. But it's human nature to view it the other way and feel you deserve a little treat for having good numbers.

The bottom line. There is no number you can reach on the glucose monitor or the bathroom scale to which I'd say, "OK, now you can eat whatever you want." Since you're going to continue choosing healthy, life-promoting foods regardless of that number, why bother with monitoring? If your number comes back high, you keep doing what you're doing, and if it comes back low, you keep doing what you are doing. In either case, that means sticking with *The 30-Day Diabetes Cure* plan. It's that simple, and it works every time.

BLOOD SUGAR BY THE NUMBERS

Be sure to read "Blood Sugar Self-Monitoring: My Recommendations May Surprise You" to understand how I'd like you to approach monitoring your blood sugar. Diabetes specialists offer these general targets:

- Normal blood sugar: Between 70 and 100 mg/dl before meals. Under 145 mg/dl two hours after a meal.

- High blood sugar: Over 140 mg/dl before a meal. Over 160 mg/dl at bedtime.

Contacting your doctor. Is there a number that should prompt you to call your doctor? Ask him or her this very question and be sure to get a clear answer.

PARTNER WITH YOUR DOCTOR ON *THE 30-DAY DIABETES CURE* PLAN

All the lab tests and glucose readings in the world are meaningless unless you work with your entire diabetes team in partnership. As you follow my plan and your body starts to reveal its astounding ability to heal your underlying condition, you should feel even more motivated to engage the experts. Here's a quick list of points to remember…

Assemble your team. Your doctor is in charge of supervising your care, and he/she may refer you to a certified diabetes educator (CDE) to help you manage monitoring, medications and lifestyle changes. Normally these educators follow the recommendations of the ADA, which fall far short of the kind of lifestyle and dietary standards you really need to reverse and heal your diabetes. By following *The 30-Day Diabetes Cure*, you'll get far better results—and faster. Your physician may also refer you to an endocrinologist who specializes in diabetes treatment. Remember that your team needs to serve you as you take charge of your own body. You are the boss, not the team.

Try a trainer. Look for a personal trainer or physical therapist with experience in diabetes who can help you with a physical fitness program. You don't necessarily need a trainer but some of my patients have found them to be very helpful and motivating. For example, Roberta discovered that lifting weights (which she'd never even considered) trimmed her up and boosted muscle strength while burning calories and improving her body's insulin sensitivity. George, a recalcitrant exerciser in his 60s, started pool exercises at his local YMCA and discovered a group of like-minded friends, which made working-out less like "work" and more like fun.

Dental do's and don'ts. Excess blood sugar feeds nasty bacteria that attack your gums. People with diabetes have more periodontal (gum) disease, and anyone with gum problems is at greater risk for heart disease. See your dentist two times a year at least, for a cleaning and a check-up, and report any gum tenderness. Don't miss flossing each and every night and don't forget to brush at least twice daily.

Share your stats. As you follow *The 30-Day Diabetes Cure*, you may want to share your success with your diabetes team. I urge you to do so. This is different than the usual obsessing over numbers. Sharing your improvements lets you take a bow for the improvements you've made which are healing your underlying diabetes. When your new way of living brings down your blood sugar, blood pressure and weight, you'll want to report this regularly. And trust me, plenty of accolades will be coming your way.

Nab a notebook. Most of us don't have perfect memories, even less so in the often-daunting environment of a doctor's office. In the days before your appointment, jot down your own list of questions, leaving a lot of empty space under each one to record your physician's answers. Ask about the tests you'll need in the months ahead and for any clarification on when and how to take your meds. Write down everything your doctor says.

Draft a dietician. You may wish to seek out a registered dietician or Nutritional Specialist if you need extra support. Give this person a copy of *The 30-Day Diabetes Cure* so he/she understands your goals. Dieticians can offer entirely practical tips and information, including where and how to shop for all the fresh, whole foods on my eating plan. They can also guide you in preparing meals if you're not particularly skillful in the kitchen.

Be wary of nutritionists who adhere to ADA dietary guidelines or who recommend ADA-approved foods, because this organization receives funding from the food giants who typically make unhealthy products. When food shopping, think "fresh and local" first. For packaged foods, learn to read ingredients closely.

Make friends with your feet. Treat them with utmost respect and care, including regular visits to a podiatrist. This foot specialist will carefully inspect your feet for numbness or tingling, cuts, cracking or sores that might be signs of delayed healing. Any signs of infection must be addressed immediately to stop progression that can lead to amputation. Your podiatrist will also check for nerve damage. Visit once a year or more as your doctor recommends. Be sure to wear your favorite shoes to the appointment. This will help your foot doctor evaluate their safety and suitability.

Eye exams are essential. According to the CDC, when a dilated eye exam discovers retina damage early, laser therapy can reduce the chances of severe vision loss by a staggering 50-60 %.[7] Schedule an annual appointment with your ophthalmologist to ensure your blood sugar isn't damaging the delicate blood vessels of your retina. If this is a new doctor for you, be certain you tell the person making the appointment that you have diabetes.

Report problems right away. Whether you experience symptoms involving your feet, skin, kidneys, circulation or eyes, it's absolutely essential to report any oddities to your doctor right away. As you follow *The 30-Day Diabetes Cure*, you'll be slowing the progression of all complications, but as you work with my plan, early detection of complications remains paramount. Tell your physician about any and all new symptoms, including numbness or tingling, pain or burning, skin changes such as cracking, dryness, or a stubborn sore, swelling or redness, a weird spot in your vision, erection difficulties, or changes in urination patterns. Don't feel embarrassed discussing any subject. Doctors are trained to listen, however personal the matter may be, and help you remedy it.

Monitor the miracle. As you work with my plan and start developing a leaner profile, a more energetic life force and improvements in your condition, honor the miracle that's happening inside you. Your pancreas is healing, your circulation is improving and your vision is clearer. Take time for meditation, prayer or a period of deep, relaxing breathing every day. Use this time to develop the attitude of gratitude.

---

[7] http://www.diabeticlivingonline.com/monitoring/doctor-visits/give-your-doctor-a-checkup/?page=2

How to Heal Your Pancreas

HOW TO HEAL YOUR PANCREAS

*"Our bodies communicate to us clearly and specifically,
if we are willing to listen to them."*

—SHAKTI GAWAIN

BY THE TIME you receive a diagnosis of type 2 diabetes, 80% of your body's ability to produce insulin may have already been destroyed. Therefore, it's essential that you learn how to protect the remaining 20%—and even increase that percentage as much as possible—so you don't spend the rest of your life injecting insulin. This means you've got to learn to love your pancreas, the organ that manufactures insulin. And to love it, you first have to get to know it.

NEED YOUR PANCREAS

The pancreas is one of the most interesting parts of the human anatomy. About an inch thick and seven inches long, it's tucked deep in the abdomen, behind your stomach. Neither a gland nor an organ, it actually behaves like both.

It's an *endocrine* gland, meaning that it secretes hormones (including insulin) into your blood; and at the same time, it's an *exocrine* gland, which means that it secretes digestive enzymes into your GI tract. Since we're primarily interested in the pancreas' insulin function, let's focus on that.

Inside your pancreas, insulin is manufactured by beta cells in the place called "islets of Langerhans" because they're organized into small islands (islets) of endocrine cells. There are about one million beta islets in a healthy adult pancreas.

THE IMPORTANCE OF INSULIN

During digestion, your body breaks down food into glucose (a simple sugar derived from the carbohydrates and starches you eat) and ensures that there's a steady supply of it for energy. Insulin assists in this process by unlocking receptor sites on the surface of your cells so glucose (blood sugar) can enter. This is the only way glucose can be metabolized into the fuel that keeps you thinking, breathing and moving.

Most people, including many doctors, believe this is insulin's main function. But insulin's primary job is making and storing fat. You see, the amount of glucose that your body can convert into energy depends upon your activity level. A marathon runner needs several thousand calories during a three-hour race and his/her metabolism is constantly converting glucose into fuel. An insufficient glucose supply will cause him/her to "hit the wall"—or run out of energy. A couch potato, on the other hand, doesn't require very much energy at all to lie on the sofa and operate the remote control.

So what happens to all of the glucose that gets converted from munching on nachos, cookies and Häagen-Dazs during an evening of prime-time TV?

HOW INSULIN RESISTANCE (PREDIABETES) OCCURS

Chowing down on the couch, unless you're replenishing the stored glucose your body used during your afternoon workout, will overload your bloodstream with blood sugar. Your body, with insulin's help, stores this energy away in the form of fat (called *triglycerides*) to be called upon during your next workout or race.

Problems start to happen when that workout or race *doesn't* happen—but the noshing continues night after night. As fat cells become more engorged, they lose their sensitivity to insulin (the condition known as *insulin resistance*) and turn away glucose, which keeps it circulating in the bloodstream. This is where your body's hormone system begins to go haywire.

Chronically elevated blood sugar sends signals to the pancreas to crank out more insulin, which creates even more fat and forces its storage. Over time, insulin finds it more and more difficult to open your cells' receptor "locks." The pancreas thinks more insulin is the solution, so it churns out yet more of the stuff. When insulin's effect becomes so weakened that the cells hardly pay attention to it, high levels of glucose remain in the bloodstream. This state is called type 2 diabetes.

FIVE VERY DANGEROUS SITUATIONS ARE NOW OCCURRING IN THE BODY

First, high levels of both glucose and insulin are now circulating through the bloodstream. Together they are highly inflammatory, as if billions of tiny shards of glass were coursing through your arteries under pressure, scratching and scraping the tissue they come in contact with. This damages the delicate lining of artery walls in the same way as if you rubbed your cheeks with sandpaper until they bled. What happens next is very much like the scabbing process that would occur on your face.

In an attempt to repair the microscopic scratches and scrapes in your arteries, your body uses fats and cholesterol to seal and heal them. Layer upon layer of these fats (called plaque) accumulate and can block arteries—or can trigger a blood clot which results in a heart attack or stroke. This is the primary reason 75% of all diabetic fatalities are caused by cardiac arrest, making it the most deadly of all complications.

Second, massive amounts of free radical molecules are generated by all this inflammation, which destroy healthy tissue—including beta cells in the pancreas. When free radical populations reach a critical mass, they overwhelm the antioxidant defense system that protects the body's DNA. Once the body's genetic blueprint is breached and damaged, cancer begins to develop. (It's especially important to note here that glucose is cancer's preferred fuel, feeding tumors just like fertilizer feeds a plant's growth.) Continuing to consume sugary carbs when you have diabetes or insulin resistance is like asking for a diagnosis of cancer.

Third, glucose molecules displace oxygen's usual (and essential) presence on red blood cells, in effect hijacking them. The result is that vital organs—among them the brain, heart, eyes, arms and legs—suffer poor circulation. This is the fundamental cause of serious diabetic complications including blindness, gangrene and limb amputation.

Fourth, without sufficient oxygen and with high levels of glucose, the blood becomes thick and slow-moving. In response, the brain sends out a "thirst signal" in an attempt to dilute the bloodstream. Gulping extra fluids (and, tragically, most diabetics reach for sugary sodas, making matters worse) causes excessive urination, and in the process the body can become dehydrated. Frequent urination also flushes out precious nutrients already in short supply, further depriving vital organs of adequate nutrition. Ultimately, the body eats its own muscle in an attempt to gain vital nutrients. This is why diabetes is called a "wasting disease."

Finally, the pancreas becomes exhausted by its overproduction of insulin, and the few remaining beta cells die. When the body can no longer produce its own insulin, a synthetic version of the hormone must be injected regularly or the patient will die. This is type 1 diabetes.

WHY DRUGS AREN'T THE SOLUTION

Drugs have the ability to lower your blood sugar count, which will make your doctor very happy. But your pancreas won't be as pleased. It will continue to wear itself out until every one of its insulin-producing beta cells is destroyed unless you improve your eating and lifestyle patterns and heal the damage that inflammation has already caused. This is what *The 30-Day Diabetes Cure* will help you achieve.

It's important to note that everyone loses beta cells as a natural part of the aging process, but for most people this loss isn't critical. However, it's a different story for a person with type 2 or insulin resistance. Scientists now know that insulin resistance is the primary killer of insulin-producing beta cells, which speeds the development of diabetes and worsen its consequences.

EATING FOR A HEALTHIER PANCREAS

One important way to help reverse diabetes and repair the damage done to your pancreas by inflammation and free radicals is to make sure your diet is rich in antioxidant foods and supplements. Simply following *The 30-Day Diabetes Cure* will cover you on both counts. Eating regular meals and snacks that contain little or no refined carbohydrates or sugar—but are loaded with fiber with adequate protein—can also keep your blood sugar levels steady without relying on glucose-lowering medications. Solid studies support this…

- Research performed at Case Western Reserve University School of Medicine in Cleveland, Ohio found that eating meals lower in refined carbs produce healthier levels of blood sugar, while reducing carbohydrate cravings. Not only does this help you control your weight without dieting, it also helps reverse insulin resistance, type 2 and a chronic sweet tooth. Once you begin *The 30-Day Diabetes Cure*, I'll explain how eating refined carbohydrate foods creates a vicious cycle of more carb craving.

- Other studies have demonstrated that consuming three regular meals a day is much better for your blood sugar and your pancreas than eating sporadically. Research published in the *European Journal of Clinical Nutrition* examined the effect that irregular meals had on glucose levels and blood fats in healthy adults. The findings confirm that people who ate irregularly had higher peak insulin levels after eating, plus elevated levels of dangerous blood fats and cholesterol afterward. The lesson here is to spread your meals and snacks evenly throughout the day—and don't skip.

HOW TO LOVE YOUR PANCREAS

If you have diabetes or prediabetes, the health of your pancreas is crucial for your survival and well-being. You'll need to love and nourish it as you would a newborn baby. You can no longer take it for granted because your life now depends upon *its* life and good health.

The 30-Day Diabetes Cure is designed so you'll naturally do all the right things for your pancreas day in and day out. You'll be protecting the beta cells you still have…doing everything science knows to undo the harm done…and, quite possibly, helping to regenerate new beta cells.

Most doctors believe it's not possible to repair a damaged pancreas, but I'm not so sure they're right. They said that about brain cells and heart cells, only to have those beliefs overturned by recent discoveries. Never underestimate the human body's remarkable ability to heal itself. Besides, there's been some promising new research indicating that the pancreas may, in fact, be able to be repaired, thus reversing diabetes naturally…

- Beta cells were able to be regenerated in laboratory animals, according to research published in 2004 in *Nature* involving Harvard scientists who clearly demonstrated it could be achieved successfully. Although similar studies have yet to be performed on humans, this is an exciting development.

- Several human studies already have shown that both weight loss and exercise can reduce insulin resistance by increasing cell sensitivity to insulin. This means that less natural insulin is required for glucose management, thereby de-stressing your beta cells and boosting their productivity and longevity.

- In 2008, the journal *Obesity* published a study examining the effect of exercise and weight loss on a group of obese, elderly adults. After just six months, their insulin sensitivity *doubled*. Losing weight and being active not only significantly lowered their odds of developing type 2 diabetes, this also increased their insulin sensitivity and improved beta cell function.

In *The 30-Day Diabetes Cure*, you'll also discover supplements that have been shown in preliminary research to enhance the function of your remaining beta cells—and perhaps even regenerate new ones.

HOW STRESS REDUCTION HEALS YOUR PANCREAS

In spite of all this promising research, most doctors still don't believe you can heal your pancreas with diet and lifestyle—or that you can heal diabetes at all. Their goal is simply to manage the disease and its symptoms with drugs.

But there's another tool that can help you heal your body and reverse your diabetes. It's called *creative visualization*. Believe it or not, your mind can actually lower your blood sugar.

It's easy to feel depressed or even desperate when you've been told you have an "incurable" medical condition such as diabetes. And when you can't get your blood sugar under control or if you begin to experience complications, your anxiety levels will surely rise. You might begin to imagine the worst and end up thwarting your healing process. Dr. Alan Jacobson at the Joslin Diabetes Center finds that many patients with diabetes experience sadness, apprehension, irritability and pessimism about their future. Patients reported that daily stress causes unpredictably low or high blood glucose levels. And they're right. Stress hormones, it turns out, tell the liver to release sugar into the blood.

Here's the good news: When patients learn stress reduction techniques such as meditation and creative visualization, they can significantly lower A1C levels, compared to patients who did not use stress reduction. Dr. Richard Surwit, PhD, author of *The Mind Body Diabetes Revolution: A Proven New Program for Better Blood Sugar Control,* has investigated the relationship between stress and glucose levels for two decades. "We've found that the effect of stress hormones on glucose metabolism is profound. So even relatively simple stress-management techniques can have clinically meaningful effects on glucose control in people with diabetes," he reports. Dr. Surwit knows that even when you try to stick with a healthy diet, get physical activity and pay attention to your glucose levels, it can still be an uphill battle to keep blood sugar under control. "In our research, we've shown that the (breathing and visualization) technique will produce a clinically significant change in blood sugar in most of the people who use it."

FOCUS ON THE POSITIVE

Most fear and anxiety we experience is based on assuming the worst, or subconsciously imagining it. With Dr. Surwit's creative visualization technique, you can turn this downward spiral of mood and blood sugar around by consciously focusing on positive outcomes when fears mount. How does it work? It's simple. Breathe deeply and visualize exactly what you need to heal in your body and practice seeing yourself whole and fully well.

Try it. Imagine your pancreas. Take a few minutes throughout the day "seeing" or visualizing your pancreas as being vibrantly pink and perfectly healthy. Actually feel millions of beta cells pumping insulin into your bloodstream and removing blood sugar. Imagine that your arteries are clean as a whistle, with your valves opening and shutting as they should. Keep those images in mind and refer to them when you feel stressed. Instead of spiking your blood sugar without even eating, you'll keep it low and controlled.

Your pancreas knows exactly what to do and will respond to the basic diabetes-reversing strategies you'll learn in *The 30-Day Diabetes Cure*. Feed it well, become more physically active and trust it to do its best job. Take a few moments throughout your day to appreciate the job it's doing. In short, love your pancreas.

Diabetes Healing Superfoods

DIABETES HEALING SUPERFOODS

DIABETES HAS GROWN to near-epidemic proportions in the United States. Nearly 24 million Americans have been diagnosed with this disease, and another 57 million people are estimated to have prediabetes. It is the seventh leading cause of death and involves serious complications such as heart disease, blindness, amputation and kidney failure. It sounds terrifying, but we have great news. There are safe, effective ways to avoid or heal diabetes and all its complications. And it's as simple as eating your next meal—especially if each meal contains some of the Top 12 Diabetes Healing Superfoods.

WHAT IS DIABETES?

Diabetes is a medical condition caused by a dysfunction in normal insulin production, which leads to a dangerous buildup of sugar (glucose) in the bloodstream. The conventional medical treatment involves various prescribed medications to reduce blood sugar, depending on the type of diabetes you have (insulin resistance, metabolic syndrome, type 1, type 2 or pregnancy-related) and how far it's progressed. Among adults with diagnosed diabetes, 16% take insulin alone to help metabolize blood sugar (usually people with type 1 diabetes whose natural insulin production mechanism is damaged), 12% take both insulin and an oral medication, 57% take oral medication only, and 15% do not take either insulin or oral medications.

Our goal is to encourage as many people as possible who already have insulin resistance, metabolic syndrome, type 2 diabetes or gestational diabetes to join the 15% who do not take medication. They can do that by managing and reversing the progression of their condition naturally. We hope that adopting the dietary concepts presented here and in *The 30-Day Diabetes Cure* will also help those with insulin-dependent type 1 reduce their need for insulin and improve their overall quality of life as well. And we *know* these foods will help with the secondary complications so often experienced by people with diabetes, such as hypertension, high or imbalanced cholesterol levels and high triglycerides that all lead to heart problems and cardiovascular disease—the primary killer of people with diabetes.

Although doctors know that what you eat directly affects your blood sugar, 85% of all people with diabetes are on some kind of medication *without* significant encouragement or a specific plan for implementing naturally healing dietary and lifestyle changes. Instead, the patient's relationship to both food and medication is based primarily on measuring blood sugar and adjusting insulin accordingly. If you eat too much sugar or carbohydrates, the medical solution is to just put more insulin in your system. Yet studies show that changing not just how much you eat but *what* you eat can improve your insulin sensitivity, protect against heart, kidney and nerve damage and actually reverse type 2 diabetes…and can help people with type 1 diabetes reduce the amount of insulin they must inject every day.

The Top 12 Diabetes Healing Superfoods have a low glycemic index and are low in calories, damaging fats and sugary, simple carbohydrates. By eating a diet rich in these foods, you can gain control over your blood-sugar levels and begin to normalize your natural insulin-producing function. Furthermore, studies show that these foods are directly associated with reducing the risk of heart disease—which is 400% greater for people with diabetes than the general population—*and* they will help you lose excess weight, which is also highly correlated with the risk of diabetes and its complications.

DISCOVER MEALS THAT HEAL

When it comes to healing diabetes, meals are your best medicine. We're talking about meals with food that's close to its natural source, food that is minimally processed, food that has its full nutritional content intact. These are the components your body needs to fuel the healing process.

To help you begin this healing process, we've included here several delicious recipes that incorporate the Diabetes Healing Superfoods. Few of these foods show up in the extremely limited "standard American diet"—but they are abundant at your neighborhood grocery store, natural foods store and local farmers' market. They are easy to prepare—and less expensive than you might think.

Recipes follow each individual Diabetes Superfood description (beginning on page 66). Give these recipes a try and you'll be well on your way to naturally moderating your blood sugar levels, losing weight naturally, and truly healing your diabetes so you can get off your medications and live a long, healthy life.

For more diabetes healing recipes—and to learn about other Diabetes Healing Superfoods— please visit our free Web site at *www.myhealingkitchen.com.*

DISCOVER FOODS THAT HEAL

THE FOODS THAT HEAL DIABETES are naturally abundant in phytonutrients such as antioxidants, essential fatty acids (EFAs), vitamins and minerals that improve insulin sensitivity, protect against blood sugar spikes and quell the systemic inflammation that leads to serious illness. This isn't like a fad diet based on eating one kind of food or nothing of another. These Superfoods are delicious and easy to incorporate into your daily diet, and they offer multiple healing benefits that not only keep blood sugar in a healthy range but also help you lose weight and ease the burden of those extra pounds on your heart.

THE TOP 12 DIABETES HEALING SUPERFOODS

1. Salmon and omega-3 seafood

2. Beans

3. Onions

4. Broccoli and other crucifers

5. Olive oil

6. Romaine lettuce

7. Yogurt

8. Grapefruit

9. Nuts

10. Curry

11. Whole grains

12. Lean meat

Let's take a close look at the individual healing properties of each of these foods, as well as the clinical studies that have proven just how powerful they really are.

CHOOSE YOUR FOODS WISELY

Glycemic Index (GI) or Glycemic Load (GL)

FOLLOW THESE SIMPLE GUIDELINES when making and enjoying diabetes healing meals:

- Choose nutrient-dense foods like whole grains, vegetables and high-quality protein.

- Reduce damaging fats.

- Eliminate starchy simple carbs like bread products.

- Avoid nutrient-poor processed foods.

By following this outline, your healing meals will keep your blood sugar at proper levels without overwhelming your insulin production. They'll also nourish and support your organs for healthy functioning.

Knowing how individual ingredients affect your blood-sugar is an important piece of this healing puzzle. If the body can't produce enough insulin to metabolize glucose as it comes into your bloodstream, it becomes a kind of slow-acting but steady poison, wreaking havoc throughout your entire body, including your blood vessels and your organs. In type 1 diabetes, there is no natural insulin production taking place in the body, so it must be injected in exactly the right amounts to avoid problems; too much is as dangerous as too little. In type 2, if excess blood sugars go unchecked long enough, the disease can eventually develop into irreversible type 1, and a life dependent on an external source of insulin.

So how do you know what to eat? In order to determine how fast carbohydrates covert to blood sugar, researchers developed the Glycemic Index (GI). *Glycemic* refers to glucose; the index refers to the amount of blood sugar in your bloodstream after you eat, so a high GI number would indicate a food that produces high blood sugar, and a low GI means a food that does not significantly raise your blood sugar.

However, scientists learned some unexpected things about food as a result of analyzing their GIs. For instance, nutritionists used to believe that all "simple" carbs like sweet desserts caused a rapid rise in blood sugar, and "complex" carbs like grains and starchy vegetables, which digest more slowly, would not cause such a rise. By measuring actual levels of blood sugar after specific carbohydrates were eaten, scientists discovered some interesting facts:

- While sweet and sugary foods do have high GIs, some starchy foods like potatoes and white bread scored higher than honey or table sugar (sucrose).

- Meats and seafood are mostly protein and fat, so they have extremely low GIs.

- Some high GI foods can be "lowered" by eating them with other low GI foods.

Diabetes-friendly foods ideally have a GI of under 50. Because GIs can be surprising, using this measurement is a helpful guide for choosing what to eat. To find out the GIs of specific foods and products, go to *www.glycemicindex.com.*

Unfortunately, there are still two problems with relying on the Glycemic Index when choosing your foods. One is that true GIs can only be determined by testing, and there a very few places that conduct these tests. That means the number of foods with proven GIs is limited. The second problem is that manufacturers are producing food combinations faster than they can be evaluated.

Also, your body's glycemic response depends on two factors: not only the type of carbohydrate you eat but also the *amount* consumed. It turns out that even if a food has a high GI, if you eat just a little of it, it won't throw your blood sugar out of whack. Thus, a new guideline was developed, the Glycemic Load (GL). In order to get a more accurate measure of food's impact on blood sugar, Dr. Walter Willett and colleagues at the Harvard School of Public Health developed this formula:

GL = (GI x Net Carbs) divided by 100
(Net Carbs are the Total Carbohydrates minus Dietary Fiber)

Low Glycemic Load foods, just like low Glycemic Index foods, help keep your blood sugar at healthy levels. So now you can control your glycemic response by consuming low-GI foods **and/or** by restricting the quantity of high GL carbohydrates. If you are diabetic, you can consume about 80 GL points a day, split evenly between meals and snacks. This offers much greater variety in food choice—but watch those portions!

You can find a great resource for nutrition information on a Web site called NutritionData. com. They have evolved a formula that estimates Glycemic Load by comparing the food's levels of commonly known nutrients and coming up with an "eGL" (Estimated Glycemic Load™) that is a reliable indicator of how a given food will affect blood sugar. In the following chapters, you will find the GI and eGL number for each of the Top 12 Diabetes Healing Superfoods, as well as an array of scientific studies about how these foods can help prevent, heal, improve and avoid the complications of diabetes.

FULLNESS FACTOR

One other consideration when choosing foods and thinking about portion control is what's called the Fullness Factor. Foods that have a high calorie to weight ratio (meaning they have few calories per gram) tend to fill you up faster. Foods that contain large amounts of fat, sugar, and/or starch like white bread have low Fullness Factors, and are much easier to overeat. Foods that contain large amounts of water, dietary fiber, and/or protein like fruit and nuts have the highest Fullness Factors. It's interesting to note how these two contrasting food groups roughly correspond to the GI and GL. We recommend that you go to NutritionData.com and do some comparisons on their easy-to-use calculators.

Now we'll look at the Top 12 Diabetes Healing Superfoods individually and discuss the excellent nutritional benefits each one offers.

OMEGA-3 SALMON AND OTHER SEAFOOD

eGL (3 ounces) = 0

WILD SALMON, RAINBOW TROUT, MACKEREL, halibut, shellfish and sardines are some of the healthiest foods on the planet, thanks to their high levels of nutritious fats. These omega-3 essential fatty acids have well-known health benefits for diabetes. They…

- Improve insulin sensitivity

- Lower triglycerides

- Reduce abnormal heart rhythms

- Lower inflammation

- Reduce blood pressure

- Improve blood clotting regulation.

Most of these benefits of omega-3 seafood are also important indicators of heart health, and diabetics have a high risk of developing—and dying from—heart disease.

OMEGA-3 LESSONS FROM THE NORTH

Scientists learned a great deal about the impact of a diet high in "fatty" fish by studying Alaskan and Greenland Inuit. These native people traditionally had a diet high in cold-water seafood as well as very low incidence of cardiovascular disease or diabetes. The Japanese, who also consume large amounts of fish, also have much lower rates of heart disease and diabetes than Americans. Conversely, since these populations began eating like modern Americans (namely, a diet high in processed foods, refined carbohydrates and damaging trans fats) and exercised less, their rates of obesity and diabetes have soared.[1]

To examine the connection between American-style eating habits, heart disease and diabetes, Dr. Sven Ebbesson of the University of Virginia studied 44 contemporary Inuit who had

---

[1] http://care.diabetesjournals.org/content/25/10/1766.full

early signs of diabetes—impaired glucose tolerance and excess weight.[2] For the study, they ate more traditional foods, especially fish and other marine animals. After four years, not a single person had advanced to type 2 diabetes.

RESOLVINS RESOLVE INFLAMMATION

Much of the diabetes-healing impact of wild salmon has to do with inflammation. Researchers at the University of California, San Diego and Switzerland's University of Fribourg discovered a connection between inflammation and diabetes.[3] Their research showed that inflammation provoked by certain immune cells called *macrophages* can lead to insulin resistance and then to type 2 diabetes. Omega-3s found in the fat of cold-water fish help your body produce anti-inflammatory *resolvins* from *eicosapentaenoic acid* (EPA) and *docosahexaenoic acid* (DHA), which also help lower blood sugar levels.

OMEGA-3s AVERT HEART PROBLEMS

If you have diabetes, you have four to five times the risk for getting heart disease than non-diabetics, so anything you can do to protect your heart is important. Part of the reason omega-3s in salmon lower heart attack rates is because they lower a fat in the bloodstream called *triglycerides*. High triglycerides contribute to metabolic syndrome, a combination of conditions that increase the risk for diabetes, stroke and cardiovascular disease. In a 6-month study of overweight adults published in the journal *Nutrition,* those who ate fish high in omega-3s were able to drop their triglyceride levels by almost 7%.[4] In another large study of more than 11,000 people with heart disease, the daily consumption of about one gram of fish oil (equivalent to a 3-ounce serving of salmon) reduced heart attacks by an amazing 45%.[5]

DIABETICS: WATCH OUT FOR WEIGHT GAIN

Excess weight is also directly linked to *insulin resistance*, because it is a very visual indication that your cells have not been metabolizing glucose properly for some time. When your glucose-overloaded cells start to resist insulin's ability to metabolize blood sugar, some of it just circulates around in your bloodstream, damaging your blood vessels and other organs; large amounts are also shuttled over to your fat cells as triglycerides. This insulin-resistance, combined with excess weight, puts you on the fast track to developing full-blown diabetes.

So the first line of defense is to learn how to manage your appetite—with the help of omega-3s —so you don't start packing on the pounds in the first place. The EPA in omega-3s stimulates

---

[2] http://stroke.ahajournals.org/cgi/content/full/39/11/3079
[3] http://www.ncbi.nlm.nih.gov/pubmed/17983584
[4] http://jn.nutrition.org/cgi/content/abstract/136/11/2766
[5] http://www.e-mfp.org/v1n2-3/fish_oil-printcopy.htm

the secretion of the hormone *leptin* that tells the brain when the stomach feels full. Without that signal—which is often chemically circumvented when you eat processed foods—it is easy to overeat. Chronic overeating leads, of course, to weight gain and obesity.

Dr. Trevor Mori at the University of Western Australia recently showed that people on a weight-loss diet that included daily consumption of omega-3 fish like salmon improved glucose and insulin metabolism.[6] People on the same diet without fish had no such improvements. Also, both groups lost the same amount of weight, but blood pressure reduction was greater among the fish eaters than the non-fish eaters. Lowering blood pressure reduces the ever-present risk of heart problems for diabetics.

NOT ALL FISH ARE FATTY-ACID FRIENDLY

Eating salmon and other omega-3 fish has huge diabetes-healing benefits, but not all omega-3 fish are healthful. Despite being rich in this diabetes-healing fat, most commercial seafoods are loaded with contaminants. Larger ocean varieties tend to be contaminated with mercury residue generated by the acid rain (created primarily by coal emissions). Since high levels of mercury have been linked to brain disorders, officials advise that pregnant women, nursing mothers, young children and women who might become pregnant avoid swordfish, shark and king mackerel, and limit their consumption of other large fish, including albacore tuna, salmon and herring.

The best fish you can eat, which is both toxin-free and has a high content of omega-3s, is wild Alaskan salmon. Regrettably, overfishing has created a shortage of these healthful, wild–caught fish, but don't be lured into choosing farmed fish instead. In fact, you should *avoid farmed fish of any kind.* They may have high levels of PCBs and chemicals from plastics, and farmed fish often contains lower amounts of healing omega-3s compared to truly wild-caught fish.

Farmed fish also have unhealthy levels of pro-inflammatory omega-6 fatty acids—an essential fat that is only useful when it is in the proper ratio to omega-3. Farmed salmon are fed excessive amounts of soy pellets instead of their natural food source; processed soy increases the ratio of omega-6 and promotes chronic inflammation in humans. Remember, inflammation is associated with insulin resistance and type 2 diabetes.

Farmed salmon also are fed large amounts of antibiotics to control diseases caused by the crowded, unnatural conditions in which they are raised. Those antibiotics get into those of us who eat the fish and impair our bodies' natural resistance to illness. Instead, choose truly wild Alaskan salmon known as chinook (also called King), sockeye, coho, chum, and pink (most of which is canned or frozen).

---

6 http://www.ajcn.org/cgi/content/full/70/5/817

FISH OIL CAPSULES: A FINE FAT

If you find it difficult to eat a lot of fish every week, consider fish oil supplements. They'll deliver the perfect amount of balanced essential fatty acids. But do fish oil capsules contain mercury and PCBs? The watchdog researchers at Consumer Labs evaluated 20 different brands and found no detectable mercury levels.[7] Almost all fish oil companies thoroughly filter their products to remove mercury residues, but check the labels to be sure, and purchase only the fish oil supplements labeled as having undergone a process called "molecular distillation," which eliminates toxins. And be certain the product you pick contains a combined minimum of 500 mg EPA and DHA, vital components of omega 3 fatty acids.

As for PCB contamination in fish oil, the Environmental Defense Fund tested 75 brands of fish oil capsules for PCB contamination and developed a Best Choice/Worst Choice list to help you choose the safest product. To see the results, go to http://www.edf.org/page. cfm?tagID=16536.

DIABETES HEALING RECIPES: WILD SALMON AND HALIBUT

Jerk Grilled Salmon with Sweet Potato Green Onion Hash Browns
Serves: 4
Prep. Time: 30 minutes (not including marinade)

Jerk seasoning is a spicy complex marinade from the Caribbean that is perfect for a hearty fish such as salmon. The sweetness of the crispy potatoes offsets the *caliente* peppers (this is a *spicy* recipe—adjust chile content according to your taste). Add a simple steamed vegetable medley to make this a filling low-calorie meal for anytime of the year.

INGREDIENTS:

Four 4 to 6 oz. salmon fillets, skin off

MARINADE:

3 green onions, chopped

4 garlic cloves, chopped

1 small onion, chopped

4 to 5 fresh Scotch bonnet or habanero chile, stemmed and seeded (wear gloves
  when handling chiles)

---

[7] www.consumerlab.com/results/omega3.asp

¼ cup fresh lime juice

2 tablespoons low-sodium soy sauce

1 tablespoon fresh thyme, chopped

2 teaspoons ground allspice

2 teaspoons black pepper

¾ teaspoon freshly grated nutmeg

½ teaspoon cinnamon

HASHBROWNS:

1 large sweet potato, peeled, shredded and rinsed in cold water

3 green onions, sliced thin

1 tablespoons pure olive oil (not extra-virgin)

1 tablespoon butter

INSTRUCTIONS:

1. Combine all marinade ingredients in a blender and puree until smooth.

2. In a shallow casserole dish or Ziploc, combine the marinade and salmon and refrigerate for an hour.

3. Heat a grill or grill pan on high heat.

4. Remove the salmon from the marinade and grill for 2 to 3 minutes on each side.

5. Heat the marinade in a small saucepan until simmering and serve as a sauce on the side.

6. Meanwhile, pan heat olive oil and butter on medium heat in a large shallow sauté pan, mix the sweet potatoes and green onions, and spread in a single layer across the bottom of the pan.

7. Allow to cook untouched for 5 to 7 minutes until the bottom forms a nice crust.

8. Flip once and allow to brown on the opposite side.

9. When potatoes are tender and both side are golden brown slide onto a plate and divide into portions. Place potatoes on the plate and salmon on top.

NUTRITION FACTS: *Calories 297.6, Total Fat 11.1g, Sat. Fat 3.4g, Cholesterol 93mg, Sodium 397.6mg, Carbs 23.5g, Fiber 4g, Sugars 5.2g, Protein 26.2g*

Halibut Scampi with Cherry Tomatoes and Green Beans
Serves: 4
Prep. Time: 20 minutes

INGREDIENTS:

1 tablespoon pure olive oil

Four 4 oz. halibut fillets, skin on

1 cup cherry tomatoes, cut in half

½ small onion, diced

4 cloves garlic, minced

1 cup white wine

½ cup fresh basil, chopped

1 tablespoon unsalted butter

1 lb. green beans, trimmed

INSTRUCTIONS:

1. Bring a large pot of water to a boil.

2. Heat the olive oil in a large sauté pan on medium high heat. Sear the fish, skin side down for 2 to 3 minutes or until skin is crispy. Remove from the pan and lower the heat to medium.

3. Saute the onions and garlic for 2 to 3 minutes. Add the wine and tomatoes and reduce for 5 minutes.

4. Add the halibut back, skin side up and continue cooking for 3 to 4 minutes more. Stir in the basil and butter.

5. While the fish is cooking, blanch the beans in the boiling water for 3 to 4 minutes.

6. Serve the fish with the beans on the side and the sauce over the top.

TIPS AND NOTES:

Try this with salmon or shrimp for some different texture and flavor. Add red chili flakes for a spicy kick.

NUTRITION FACTS: *Calories 251.7, Total Fat 7.6g, Sat. Fat 2.3g, Cholesterol 48mg, Sodium 89.2mg, Carbs 13.5g, Fiber 4.9g, Sugars 0g, Protein 25.9g*

BEANS KEEP BLOOD SUGAR IN CHECK

eGL (1 cup) = 14

BEANS ARE OUR FAVORITE SUPERFOOD in the Diabetes Healing Diet because of how well they regulate blood sugar. Since they break down into glucose slowly, they don't overwhelm the body's insulin response, and their high protein and low calorie content make them a valuable helper for losing or preventing the excess weight that is so dangerous for people with diabetes.

BEANS ARE GLUCOSE SLOW-POKES

Beans rank low on the Glycemic Index (GI) (under 50 for most varieties) which means they break down into glucose slowly in the bloodstream, as opposed to high GI foods like white bread or soda. A slow entry into the bloodstream gives the body's natural insulin response adequate time to usher that glucose along at its appropriate pace, rather than being overwhelmed by a rush of sugars, which creates insulin resistance and eventually results in diabetes. In a five-year study of 64,000 women, reported by the *American Journal of Clinical Nutrition*, eating beans regularly resulted in a 38% reduction in risk for type 2 diabetes.[8]

Not only are beans low GI, they actively control blood sugar. The same pigments that give nutrient-dense berries their color are also present in beans, and those pigments are actually an antioxidant polyphenol called *anthocyanin*. Anthocyanins help control blood sugar and limit the damage diabetes causes to blood and arteries. Adding just three cups of beans per week to your diet—that's about one bean burrito, one serving of bean soup, and one serving of three-bean salad—can significantly improve your blood sugar and reduce your risk of developing diabetes, especially if you substitute beans for high GI refined carbohydrates like noodles, bread, and white rice.

REDUCE INSULIN DEPENDENCE WITH BEANS

For people who already have diabetes, beans can reduce your need for insulin medications. Dr. James Anderson of the Human Nutrition Research Center of the USDA was one of the early research pioneers on the health benefits of fiber, and he found that people with type 1 diabetes were able to reduce their need for insulin by 44% just by eating beans. And for those with type 2 diabetes, eating beans not only reduced their need for insulin and other diabetic medications, but in some cases all but eliminated the need for supplemental insulin.[9]

---

[8] http://www.naturalhealthresearch.org/nhri/?p=76
[9] http://www.ars.usda.gov/main/site_main.htm?modecode=12-35-00-00

BEANS ARE RIGHT FOR THE DIABETES WAISTLINE

People with diabetes often struggle with weight, especially with dangerous belly fat. Beans are high in protein and low in calories, making them an ideal ally in the weight-loss efforts of people with diabetes. Eating beans instead of meat at several meals a week can lower your fat and calorie intake, thus helping you drop excess pounds (and helping you manage your budget, as well). In a recent study conducted by researchers at the University of Southern California, overweight Latino children—a population with a much greater incidence of being overweight and diabetic than the general US population—substituted a half cup of beans for one daily soda. They were able to lower their risk for type 2 diabetes, reduce their weight and enjoy a significant improvement in insulin response.

Because of this slow transition of bean's carbohydrates into sugars in your bloodstream, beans assist your body's insulin response to glucose and help you burn fat faster. An Australian study found that for those people who ate meals composed of a mere 5% resistant starch, such as beans, the rate at which their bodies burned fat increased by an amazing 23% for 24 hours afterward.

FABULOUS FIBER FOUND IN BEANS

Beans also are high in soluble fiber, which binds to carbohydrates and slows their digestion into the bloodstream, preventing wild swings in blood sugar levels. They also contain generous amounts of resistant starch, which means that beans are less digestible than other carbs in the small intestine, so they move into the large intestine faster. Once there, they behave like a dietary fiber, limiting the sharp rise of glucose levels and insulin that can follow a meal.

BEANS OPEN INSULIN DOORWAYS

Another great benefit of eating beans is their high pectin content. Pectin and other fibers in beans help sensitize your cells to insulin and aid in its uptake by producing extra insulin-receptors on the cells. These insulin-receptors function as "doorways" that make it easier for insulin to do its two-fold job of removing glucose from the blood and ushering it into the cells where it's used as the body's essential fuel.

SO MANY DIABETES HEALING BEANS TO CHOOSE FROM

Beans are part of the legume family, which includes lentils, split peas, string beans, as well as all the dry beans like pinto and red beans, offering a cornucopia of colors, textures and recipe possibilities. Black beans and red kidney beans top the list for total dietary fiber and resistant starch. Lentils and chickpeas rate very low on the Glycemic Index, making them the stars of the legume family in terms of stabilizing blood sugars. Whether it's a three-bean salad, baked beans, boiled beans, refried beans, bean soup or bean dip—beans cook up in endless ways. All these bean dishes are packed with healthy fiber, which will help you control and stabilize your blood sugar levels and keep your weight down.

DIABETES HEALING RECIPE: BEANS

Chicken Cassoulet
Serves: 8 to 10
Prep. Time: 2 days

Don't be intimidated by the slightly lengthy process for this dish. It's a classic for a reason, adapted and perfected throughout France across the ages. This version combines the traditional healing white beans and onion but substitutes the usual duck confit and pork belly with lower fat poultry versions. If you don't have two days, you can broil for the last fifteen minutes to get the crispy crust, although the flavors won't be as deep or developed. Ask your friends as they gobble it up…it's worth the time and effort.

INGREDIENTS:

4 chicken thighs

½ lb. ground chicken or turkey

½ lb. lowfat turkey bacon, cut into large chunks

2 white onions, 1 quartered and 3 chopped

6 cloves garlic, 4 smashed, 2 minced

1 bay leaf

2 sprig thyme

1 sprig parsley

4 cups cooked white beans (tarbais, cannellini or navy)

1 tablespoon pure olive oil

2 to 3 cups low sodium chicken broth

INSTRUCTIONS:

1. Preheat the oven to 375 degrees F.

2. Bake the chicken thighs in a shallow casserole dish for 25 to 35 minutes. Remove from the oven and cool.

3. In a medium sauté pan, cook the ground chicken, 2 cloves minced garlic, bay leaf, 1 sprig of thyme and parsley for 5 to 7 minutes or until cooked through. Add ¼ cup water and cook 1 to 2 minutes more. Remove the meat from the pan. Add the bacon, onion, smashed garlic, and rest of thyme, and brown for 7 to 10 minutes.

4. Transfer the onion mixture to a blender and mix until smooth.

5. When the chicken thighs are cool, remove the skin and shred the meat into medium sized pieces.

6. Layer the ingredients in a deep, lightly oiled casserole dish. Start with a layer of beans, then shredded chicken, then beans, then ground chicken (remove bay leaf), etc. Spread a thin spoonful of the pureed onion mixture between each layer and finish with beans on the top.

7. Pour enough chicken broth to just cover the beans. Reserve ¼ cup broth.

8. Bake the cassoulet in a 350 degree oven for one hour. Reduce the heat to 250 degrees and cook for another hour. Cool and refrigerate overnight.

9. The next day, preheat the oven to 350 degrees and cook for another hour. Lower the oven to 250 degrees, break the crust with a spoon and add ¼ cup of the reserved liquid. Bake for another fifteen minutes or until hot throughout.

TIPS AND NOTES:

Substitute duck, beef or a medley of vegetables such as eggplant, sweet peppers, carrots and parsnips for the chicken. If using vegetables, reduce the cooking time by half so they don't turn into mush. Tie the herbs together with butchers twine before adding to the bean liquid so they are easier to get out and discard.

> **NUTRITION FACTS:** *Serving Size 227g, Calories 547, Total Fat 13.4g, Sat. Fat 3.7g, Cholesterol 61mg, Sodium 499mg, Carbs 65.4g, Fiber 16.1g, Sugars 4g, Protein 41.9g*

ONIONS FIGHT DIABETES

eGL (1 cup) = 5

ONIONS AND THEIR CLOSE COUSINS—garlic, chives, scallions, shallots and leeks—are valuable allies in the fight against diabetes because they help lower blood sugar levels, increase sensitivity to insulin, and prevent diabetic complication such as heart disease and stroke. Packed with phytonutrients, they are a good source of beneficial vitamin C, contain no fat and are loaded with dietary fiber.

ONIONS FREE UP INSULIN

Onions lower glucose levels in people with diabetes due to the curious role of one of its phytonutrients, the sulfur compound *allyl propyl disulfide*, or APDS. Since insulin is also a disulfide, APDS competes with it to occupy sites in the liver where insulin is deactivated. By blocking the breakdown of insulin in the liver, the amount of free insulin available to the body is increased. This is good news for people with diabetes, because the more insulin available to usher glucose into the cells where it can be used as your body's fuel, the lower the glucose levels in the bloodstream. Onion's cousin, garlic, is also a powerful food for lowering blood sugar, as well as helping to repair the pancreas and stimulating it to produce insulin.

FIND THE *FLAVONOIDS* IN ONIONS

Onions and garlic have positive cardiovascular effects because they are a rich source of dietary flavonoids, a class of plant compounds known for their antioxidant activity. (Antioxidants play an important role by scavenging for free radicals that can damage the body's cells, tissue, organs, and eventually, entire systems.) Researchers at Cornell University found that flavonoids such as those found in onions are associated with a reduced risk for cancer, heart disease and diabetes.

Onions, especially onion skins, contain the potent antioxidant flavonoid called quercetin, which helps protect against the eye problems associated with diabetes, especially retinopathy. The amount of quercetin your body absorbs from onions is more than 300% greater than that of apples and twice what you get from tea. UK researchers estimate that onions contain between 22-52 mg of quercetin per medium-sized onion, and that the daily consumption of onions increases the accumulation of quercetin in the blood. The next time you make soup, consider leaving the onion skin on.

GET A CHROMIUM BOOST FROM ONIONS

Onions are also very high in chromium, a trace mineral essential for metabolizing glucose and helping promote insulin sensitivity. Some studies show that eating foods rich in chromium, such as onions, helps decrease fasting blood glucose levels, improve glucose tolerance and decrease total cholesterol and triglycerides.

According to biophysiologist and nutritionist, Dr. Kurt D. Grange, Ph.D., chromium levels naturally decrease with age. However, chromium deficiency may already be a widespread problem in the US, since the body's reserves of chromium are depleted by consuming refined sugar and white flour and by insufficient exercise. Chromium deficiency can lead to glucose intolerance, obesity and Type 2 diabetes. Only one cup of onions supplies 20% of your daily chromium needs.

DIABETES CRIES FOR ONIONS

In general, the milder the onion's flavor, the less potent it is as a healing food for diabetes. Researchers at both the University of Wisconsin and Cornell University found that the more pungent the onion, the more health benefits you'll receive in terms of anti-platelet activity, which keeps blood cells less "sticky" so they don't clump together and form clots (which can cause as heart attack or stroke). So chop up those onions and weep with joy at the diabetes-healing power you are about to put in your meal.

DIABETES HEALING RECIPE: ONIONS

Rosemary Mushroom Bolognese Stew with White Beans
Serves: 4
Prep. Time: 45 minutes

On a warm winter night in front of the fire, there is nothing better than to snuggle up with a good book and big bowl of piping hot soup. A vegetarian version of the classic meat pasta combines woody mushrooms, protein-packed white beans and bright tomatoes to create a healthy starch-free meal. Serve this with a simple green salad and the meal is complete.

INGREDIENTS:

1 tablespoon pure olive oil

1 white onion, peeled and diced

1 carrot, peeled and diced

1 celery stalk, peeled and diced

2 cloves garlic, minced

1 lb. mushrooms, (button, shiitake, porcini, chanterelle, Portobello) cleaned and diced

½ cup red wine

1 cup canned diced tomatoes, with juice

3 cups low sodium vegetable or chicken stock

2 cups cooked white beans

1 sprig fresh rosemary

1 bay leaf

INSTRUCTIONS:

1. In a large stockpot, heat the olive oil on medium heat.
2. Saute the onion, carrot and celery for 4 to 5 minutes or until they start to soften.
3. Add the garlic and mushroom and cook for 5 minutes more, stirring often.
4. When the mushrooms start to release their liquid, turn the heat to high and add the wine. Cook on high heat for 3 to 4 minutes or until wine is almost evaporated.
5. Add the tomatoes, chicken stock, cooked beans, bay leaf and rosemary and lower heat to a simmer.
6. Cook for 20 to 30 minutes or until all vegetable are soft and liquid is reduced to desired consistency (cook longer for a thicker stew).
7. Remove the rosemary sprig and bay leaf and garnish with the grated cheese.

TIPS AND NOTES:

Add a small amount of lean ground bison to make this an even heartier soup. You can also substitute the white beans for black or pinto and add some jalapenos and cilantro to give this dish a southwestern flavor.

> **NUTRITION FACTS:** *Calories 279, Total Fat 4.3g, Sat. Fat 0.6g, Cholesterol 0mg, Sodium 148.4mg, Carbs 44.5g, Fiber 10.6g, Sugars 4.3g, Protein 14.3g*

BROCCOLI BEATS DIABETES COMPLICATIONS

eGL (1 cup) = 3

BROCCOLI IS ONE OF THE MOST POWERFUL diabetes healing foods on earth, thanks to its plentiful array of vitamins, minerals, fiber and especially antioxidants that help prevent damage from free radicals. Broccoli boosts your immune system and helps you avoid diabetes and all its complications, especially cardiovascular disease.

SAVE YOUR DIABETIC HEART WITH *SULFORAPHANE*

People with diabetes are four to five times as likely to develop cardiovascular diseases such as heart attack or stroke. The key healing compound in broccoli is *sulforaphane*, which plays a major role in protecting damaged blood vessels. Too much glucose in the bloodstream eventually damages and constricts the blood vessels, which is also why people with diabetes suffer from circulation problems in their feet, lower legs and hands. But according to the Mayo Clinic, sulforaphane encourages the production of enzymes that reduce the blood vessel damage triggered by high blood sugar levels, thus helping to minimize the devastating effects of diabetes.

According to a study by UK researchers published in the journal *Diabetes*, the sulforaphane in broccoli not only helps boost your immune system and support the liver's job of detoxifying your body, it also protects against oxidative stress. Oxidative stress is a term for the damage done to cells, tissues and blood vessels by Reactive Oxygen Species (ROS) molecules, which include free radicals. The sulforaphane in broccoli activates a protein in the body called *nrf2*, which switches on genes that increase the body's production of its own antioxidants and detoxifying enzymes. In lab tests, sulforaphane was found to double the activation of the protein nrf2 and to reduce ROS molecules by an astonishing 73%.

All of broccoli's cruciferous cousins contain sulforphane, including kale, cabbage, collards, bok choy, mustard greens, kohlrabi, turnips, cauliflower, arugula and watercress. If you don't like broccoli or its cousins, try a wrap with broccoli sprouts, which have the very highest concentrations of sulforaphane.

BROCCOLI'S VITAMIN C FIGHTS FREE RADICALS

Broccoli has additional diabetes-healing power with its high levels of vitamin C. Because the body can't manufacture vitamin C, we must get it from the food we eat. One cup of broccoli delivers about 116 milligrams of this powerful antioxidant, almost twice the minimum recommended daily amount for adults. According to the Linus Pauling Institute, vitamin C even in small amounts can protect against the damage done by free radicals and oxidative stress that results from exposure to pollution, toxins and an unhealthy diet—damage that can lead to directly to diabetes, cardiovascular disease or stroke.

A sixteen year study, published in the *Journal of the American College of Cardiology*, involving 1500 women with diabetes found that supplementation with 400mg or more of vitamin C each day significantly reduced the risk of coronary heart disease. Also, a team of scientists from Harold Hamm Diabetes Center in Oklahoma and the University Hospital of Coventry discovered that a combined therapy of insulin and highly controlled levels of vitamin C stopped disease-related blood vessel damage in patients with type 1 diabetes.

INSULIN RECEPTORS LOVE CRUCIFER'S CHROMIUM

Like onions, broccoli is a great source of the trace mineral chromium, used to manufacture the glucose tolerance factor, or GTF, which helps break down blood sugar. According to the Linus Pauling Institute, the chromium in broccoli helps lower your blood sugar, cholesterol and triglycerides, which greatly reduces your risk of diabetes and cardiovascular disease. Chromium aids in the metabolism of glucose by re-sensitizing the insulin receptors on the surface of every cell. Many Americans are chromium-deficient because a diet heavy in refined carbohydrates such as white sugar and white flour is not only low in chromium, it also depletes chromium from your body.

FIND THE FIBER TO FIGHT DIABETES

Dietary fiber is the roughage that makes you feel full without gaining weight, and broccoli is loaded with it. Foods that are high in fiber help slow the metabolism of glucose and control blood sugar levels, thus reducing your risk of developing diabetes or cardiovascular disease. High fiber foods such as broccoli also support weight loss, which helps to lower insulin resistance. The fewer cells resist insulin, the more insulin can usher glucose into your body's cells.

BETA-CAROTENE—THE EYES HAVE IT

One of the complications of diabetes is retinopathy, which causes a slow loss of vision. Broccoli is rich in *beta-carotene*, which your body uses to make vitamin A, another powerful antioxidant that is necessary for healthy eyes. When selecting broccoli, choose those stalks with the darkest color, because that means it has the most beta-carotene. Eat it raw or lightly cooked and don't forget to eat both the stems and leaves. The stems are not only sweet and mild-flavored, they're much higher in fiber than the broccoli florets, and the leaves are the richest source of beta-carotene.

COOK BROCCOLI WITH CARE

Preserve broccoli's diabetes healing nutrients by eating it raw, lightly steamed or sautéed. Raw broccoli can be chopped and added to salads, sandwiches or even green smoothies. Overcooking destroys its nutrients; a minute or two in the microwave with a small amount of water is all you need to give broccoli a crisp finish. Drizzle with extra-virgin olive oil or a small pat of butter and sprinkle with sesame seeds for a crunchy treat. (See also pages 98–100 for a diabetes-healing recipe that incorporates broccoli.)

OLIVE OIL HELPS MANAGE DIABETES

eGL (1 cup) = 0

OLIVE OIL IS A SUPERFOOD for many medical conditions, but is especially important in the Diabetes Healing Diet. A diet rich in olive oil has enhanced the health of Mediterranean peoples for thousands of years, making it a time-tested—as well as highly researched—ally for people with diabetes. It helps stabilize blood sugar levels and prevent diabetic complications such as stroke and heart disease.

OLIVE OIL LOWERS GLUCOSE

Olive oil is one of the *monounsaturated fats*, which are especially important for people with diabetes because they help control glucose levels. Many nutritionists believe that people with diabetes should eat a low-fat/low-carb diet—low in fat to help prevent heart damage, and fewer carbohydrates to avoid severe swings in blood sugar levels. But new research finds that a diet rich in monounsaturated fats such as olive oil is even more effective in controlling diabetes. A study published in the journal of the German Diabetes Association found that glucose levels were lower in people who ate monounsaturated fats than those who avoided all fats.

GOOD FAT = GOOD CHOLESTEROL

Olive oil also helps lower cholesterol. The same researchers also found that the monounsaturated fats present in olive oil helped lower LDL ("bad") cholesterol, keep triglyceride levels in check, and increase HDL ("good") cholesterol. This is important information for people with diabetes, because cardiovascular disease is one of its most serious complications. Doctors often prescribe medication to balance cholesterol and lower triglycerides, so eating olive oil regularly is an effective way to reduce your need for so many pills.

LOSE WEIGHT, MEDITERRANEAN STYLE

Surprisingly, olive oil helps you lose weight. Researchers in Spain concluded that a calorie-controlled diet high in monounsaturated fat such as olive oil did not cause weight gain among people with diabetes, an important consideration because excess weight exacerbates the disease. They also found that including olive oil was more realistic (and pleasing) than eating a strict low-fat diet. Anyone who's tried a strict diet knows that it only works if you're able to stick with it.

HIGH QUALITY FOR HIGH HEALING

Eating the highest quality olive oil you can afford is important in order to obtain all its diabetes-healing nutrients. Extra virgin olive oil has the most benefits because it's from the first pressing of the olives. Best when unfiltered, olive oil should have a deep golden yellow to dark green color and come in a dark bottle (or be stored in a dark pantry). Choose cold-pressed, which means it was not processed with heat or chemicals (both of which can destroy this delicate oil's nutritional value).

DIABETES HEALING RECIPE: OLIVE OIL

Garlic Hummus
Serves: 4-6
Prep. Time: 10 minutes

This easy, versatile spread combines a trio of diabetes-fighting ingredients to control glucose, stimulate insulin production and lower cholesterol. Beans, garlic and extra virgin olive oil are not only tasty but filled with antioxidants and vitamins that promote weight loss and diabetes health.

INGREDIENTS:

1 can garbanzo beans, drained and rinsed

2 tablespoons lemon juice

4 to 8 cloves garlic

¼ cup extra virgin olive oil

INSTRUCTIONS:

Combine all ingredients in a food processor or blender and blend until desired consistency. Hummus can be as smooth or as chunky as you like.

TIPS AND NOTES:

Serve this super simple healing dip with fresh vegetables and low-carb spelt crackers or as a spread on a low carb pita with tomato slices, red onion, lettuce, cucumber and a dollop of low-fat yogurt. For a true Mediterranean feast, combine this zesty hummus with quinoa tabouli and roasted eggplant baba ganoush.

NUTRITION FACTS: *Calories 179.5, Total Fat 9.9g, Sat. Fat 1.3g, Cholesterol 0mg, Sodium 240.7mg, Carbs 19.3g, Fiber 3.6g, Sugars 0g, Protein 4.1g*

ROMAINE LETTUCE HEALS DIABETES

eGL (1 cup) = 1

NOT ALL LETTUCE IS CREATED EQUAL. Romaine lettuce is far superior to its popular rival, iceberg lettuce, when it comes to vitamins, minerals, phytonutrients and dietary fiber—all necessary for people with diabetes. Romaine lettuce—and similar nutrient-rich lettuces like red leaf and green leaf—helps metabolize glucose and stabilize blood sugar levels, combats the damaging oxidation done by free radicals and helps prevent heart disease.

CHROMIUM CALMS DIABETES

Romaine lettuce and other leafy greens are rich in chromium, an essential mineral your body uses to manufacture the *glucose tolerance factor* (GTF) in order to break down blood sugar and keep it from accumulating in your bloodstream. According to the Linus Pauling Institute, chromium works by re-sensitizing the insulin receptors on the surface of every cell. Chromium not only helps lower your blood sugar, it lowers cholesterol and triglycerides as well, which helps reduce your risk of developing metabolic syndrome, the precursor to diabetes. Refined carbohydrates such as white sugar and white flour are not only low in chromium, they deplete it from your body. No wonder many Americans are chromium-deficient. Two cups of Romaine lettuce contains 13% of your daily nutritional value (DNV) of chromium.

ROMAINE PROMOTES INSULIN SENSITIVITY

Low-calorie romaine lettuce is packed with dietary fiber. Remember that eating unprocessed, high-fiber foods is essential for people with diabetes because they help slow the metabolism of glucose, increase insulin sensitivity and stabilize blood sugar levels. Dietary fiber-rich foods such as romaine lettuce also help your body eliminate toxins, lower high cholesterol and lose weight. Four low-cal veggie wraps made with four big leaves of crunchy romaine will give you up to 8% of your DNV for dietary fiber.

ROMAINE'S DIABETES HEALING SUPER-HEROES

Here's the special diabetes healing power you'll get with a salad made with two cups of romaine:

35% of your DNV for manganese. Manganese is a mineral that aids in the metabolism of fats and carbohydrates, and romaine is full of it. Manganese is a component of manganese superoxide dismutase, or Mn-SOD, an antioxidant which scavenges for free radicals and repairs the damage they cause. Manganese also helps protect against the oxidation of LDL (bad) cholesterol, preventing the buildup of plaques in the arteries, which can lead to atherosclerosis, cardiovascular disease and stroke.

According to researchers at the University of Maryland, as many as 37% of Americans are manganese-deficient. Why? Because refined foods are deficient in this essential mineral. Interestingly, some research has found that people with diabetes have much lower levels of manganese than normal, but it is unknown whether this is a cause or an effect of diabetes. Add some summer squash, green beans, mushrooms and brown rice to your romaine lettuce and you'll have almost all the manganese you need.

60% of your DNV for vitamin A. Romaine lettuce is extremely high in the pro-vitamin A carotenoid, beta-carotene. Beta-carotene is important in healing diabetic complications like cardiovascular disease and stroke because it helps stop LDL (bad) cholesterol from forming into artery-blocking plaques. Add a quarter cup of grated carrots to your salad and you'll top 100%.

Need More? Romaine lettuce and other leafy greens like spinach are an excellent source of the antioxidant *lutein*, another carotenoid which the body coverts into *zeaxanthin*. Lutein not only neutralizes oxidative damage done by free radicals and helps prevent atherosclerosis, but, according to a study published by the *Journal of the Science of Food and Agriculture,* it also helps improve eye health. This is important for people with diabetes, who are at much greater risk for developing *retinopathy*, cataracts and macular degeneration.

45% of your DNV for vitamin C. Romaine's antioxidant vitamin C scavenges for free radicals and prevents the damage they do to blood vessels. The team of vitamin K, vitamin C plus beta-carotene helps prevent cholesterol from becoming oxidized and sticky, which makes it build up in your arteries to form damaging plaques.

140% of your DNV for vitamin K. Vitamin K also prevents arterial plaque and may also improve insulin resistance. In a recent 3 year study published in *Diabetes Care*, researchers found that vitamin K decreased insulin resistance in men over sixty.

38% of your DNV for folate. Romaine lettuce and other leafy greens are high in *folic acid,* a B vitamin which helps lower high blood pressure and prevent damage to blood vessels, thereby reducing the risk of heart attack and stroke. In a study of more than 150,000 women, those who consumed folic acid such as that found in romaine lettuce were able to significantly decrease their risk of high blood pressure and the cardiovascular disease which can develop as a result.

ROMAINE LETTUCE UNLIMITED

This extraordinary lettuce need not be limited to salads. You can use romaine leaves in place of bread or tortillas to make a low-calorie "wrap," or layer it on to reduce the amount of meat in your sandwich. You can even add lettuce leaves to your favorite fruit smoothie, dramatically increasing its nutritional value and amount of healthy dietary fiber.

GO GREEN WITH ROMAINE

Local produce is always more nutritious. Industrially grown lettuce, even if it's touted as organic, is often transported over long distances, sometimes halfway around the world. It's washed with chlorine and often treated with other chemicals to prolong its shelf-life. While these practices may benefit the big industrial grower and vendor, they don't do much for your health. Instead, consider supporting the growers at your local farmer's market; they make every effort to differentiate their growing practices from those of big agribusiness. And the lettuce and greens you buy locally will taste better and be healthier for you because they'll be much fresher. You can take even more control of your health by growing lettuce yourself.

DIABETES HEALING RECIPE: ROMAINE LETTUCE

Braised Romaine and Cipollini Onions in Stout Beer with Crushed Walnuts
Serves: 4 to 6
Prep. Time: 30 minutes

This is a perfect winter side dish that warms the tummy without adding pounds. By reducing the easy sauce of beer and stock with just a touch of balsamic you can get the feel of a nice thick glaze without the added sugar. Soft sweet onions add a bite, and the crunch of walnuts at the end brings it all together.

INGREDIENTS:

2 teaspoons pure olive oil

2 cloves garlic, minced

¼ to ½ teaspoon red chili flakes (more or less to taste)

¾ lb. cipollini onions, peeled and halved

½ cup stout beer

1 cup low sodium chicken broth

1 tablespoon balsamic vinegar

1 tablespoon Dijon mustard

2 heads romaine lettuce, cut in quarters lengthwise

GARNISH:

2 tablespoons walnuts, toasted and crushed

INSTRUCTIONS:

1. In a large sauté pan, heat the olive oil on medium heat.

2. Add the garlic and red chili flakes and sauté for 1 minute, stirring constantly.

3. Add the onions, beer, chicken stock, vinegar and mustard and bring to a low simmer.

4. Cook for 20 to 25 minutes or until onions are tender and sauce is reduced by half.

5. Add the romaine, cover and cook for 3 to 5 minutes more.

6. Remove the lettuce while the center is still firm and the leaves are just wilted.

7. Turn the heat up to reduce the sauce to a glazelike consistency.

8. Curl the romaine on the plate and pour the onions and sauce over. Garnish with the crushed walnuts.

> **NUTRITION FACTS:** *Calories 78.2, Total Fat 3.4g, Sat. Fat 0.4g, Cholesterol 0mg, Sodium 82.4mg, Carbs 8.6g, Fiber 2.5g, Sugars 0.4g, Protein 2.7g*

YOGURT TO PREVENT AND HEAL DIABETES

eGL (1 cup) = 10

Yogurt is known for its "good bacteria" that help digestion, but the important news for diabetics is that yogurt improves glucose metabolism, insulin sensitivity, high blood pressure and cholesterol. The beneficial bacteria are *probiotics*, which means "for life," and yogurt truly is a diabetic's life healer.

YOGURT IS LIVING AND LIFE-GIVING

One reason yogurt is such a dynamic healer is because it's a living food, the result of adding beneficial bacteria to milk and keeping it warm until the lactose, or milk sugar, turns to lactic acid and ferments. This provides the perfect breeding ground for these "good" bacteria so they can multiply. So eating live yogurt regularly is like sending in the cavalry to reinforce the beneficial bacteria in your GI tract. These beneficial bugs represent one way in which nature keeps the "bad guy" bacteria (such as e. coli, salmonella, listeria, campylobacter, and clostridium perfringens, which cause food poisoning and other health problems) from overwhelming your body and challenging your immune system. For the best diabetes-healing power, make sure your yogurt has *Lactobacillus* and *Bifidobacterium,* which give yogurt its characteristic lemony taste.

PROBIOTICS: DEFENDING DIGESTION

Insulin resistance prevents nutrients from passing across cell membranes, so people with diabetes have cells that are actually being starved of nutrition. Probiotic bacteria in yogurt—along with lactose, protein, calcium, magnesium and potassium—slow the digestion of food sugars so that they don't assault the blood stream. A study of 3,000 people found that those who were overweight but ate dairy foods like yogurt were 70% less likely to develop insulin resistance (a precursor to diabetes) than those who didn't.

YUMMY YOGURT HELPS WITH WEIGHT

The link between being overweight and having diabetes is undeniable; 85% of type 2 diabetics are overweight. When a person is overweight, the cells in the body become less sensitive to the insulin that is released from the pancreas. Yogurt can help. According to a study published in the *International Journal of Obesity*, when obese men and women ate three six-ounce servings of fat-free yogurt daily while on a reduced-calorie diet, they lost 22% more weight and shed 80% more abdominal fat than those who ate the same number of calories, but got only one serving of dairy products. The yogurt-eaters lost an impressive 61% more body fat than the non-yogurt group.

YOGURT LOWERS BLOOD PRESSURE

Diabetics have another reason to add probiotic yogurt to their daily diet. High blood sugar causes plaque build-up in arteries, increasing the risk for high blood pressure (hypertension), heart attack and stroke. In several large studies, including one that involved 12,550 adults, the development of type 2 diabetes was 2.5 times more likely in those with hypertension. And it's a double whammy because once you have type 2 diabetes, you're twice as likely to also have hypertension. This affects 30% of type 1 diabetes patients, too.

Anti-hypertensive drugs don't always work for hypertensive diabetes—sometimes they even aggravate the problem. However, a research report from Denmark published in the *European Journal of Clinical Nutrition* notes that lactobacillus bacteria significantly lowered blood pressure in men and women after just eight weeks. The consumption of probiotics, like those in yogurt, is a new therapeutic strategy for diabetics with high blood pressure.

A LITTLE YOGURT FOR A LOT OF GOOD CHOLESTEROL

Insulin resistance, the precursor to full-blown diabetes, often leads to increased by high levels of LDL "bad" cholesterol. According to a clinical trial published in the *European Journal of Clinical Nutrition,* women who eat yogurt every day may experience as much as 38% increase in the level of "good" cholesterol. High HDL is associated with heart health. Medical studies in Japan and Argentina also found that lactobacillus bacteria found in yogurt lowered total blood cholesterol by 22% and triglycerides by 33%. Did they have to eat huge quantities of yogurt? Not at all. All it took was 3 ounces of plain yogurt a day, half of a little container from the grocery store. But be sure your yogurt contains *Lactobacillus* and *Bifidobacterium* and no added sugars.

PROBIOTICS ARE BEST FOR BETA CELLS

In an article in *Diabetologia,* scientists demonstrated that probiotics also protect beta cells in the pancreas. When healthy, these cells create and secrete insulin to digest sugars. When unhealthy, they provoke an autoimmune response causing the pancreas to self-destruct, which can lead to Type 1 insulin-dependent diabetes. Another study reported in the *Journal of Clinical Endocrinology and Metabolism* shows promising new evidence that the body has some ability to regenerate damaged beta cells, prevent the onset of insulin-dependent diabetes, and help Type 1 diabetics recover some insulin secretion ability. These powerful probiotic bacteria need to be replenished regularly, so make yogurt a part of your daily diet.

MIRCROFLORA COOL INFLAMMATION

By eating yogurt every day, you fill your digestive with "natural intestinal gut microflora." High levels of microflora have been associated with lower levels of systemic inflammation. A study in the *World Journal of Gastroenterology* found that the probiotics in yogurt trigger a decrease in C-reactive protein (CRP), the blood marker for inflammation. This is important because numerous studies have shown an association between insulin-resistance in type 2 diabetes and chronic low-grade inflammation. Try cooling your "inflamed" diabetes with a yogurt smoothie or a bowl of blueberries and yogurt.

A breakthrough paper published in *Nature* in December 2006 reported that microbial populations in the gut are different between obese and lean people. Also, bacterial populations in the gut of diabetics differ from non-diabetics, says a new study from Denmark. When microbes have abnormalities, type 2 diabetes can be the result. Probiotics affect these microbes in a positive way. A researcher from Imperial College London of Imperial said probiotics "talk" with the gut microbes and improve digestion.

GET THE BEST DIABETES HEALING YOGURT

Yogurt is one of the few probiotic foods that Americans regularly eat. But not all yogurts are equal. Many store-bought products can be loaded with sugar, artificial flavors and additives that are not good for you. Check the package to make sure you are getting the benefits of active Diabetes Healing probiotics: *Lactobacillus* and *Bifidobacterium*.

The very best yogurt for diabetics is Greek yogurt because the whey has been removed to create a thicker consistency. Whey is mostly lactose and it can spike insulin levels in people with type 2 diabetes as well as in healthy people, according to a research report last year in *The American Journal of Clinical Nutrition*. Insulin spikes make us hungry, which may make us gain weight—which increases the risk of diabetes. Greek yogurt is higher in protein, which digests more slowly.

To be certain you get the most effective healing micro-organisms in your yogurt, it's best to make your own at home. We tested several yogurt making methods…Although all methods are successful, the thermos method is the easiest of all and a foolproof way to keep the batch warm while it ferments. Just pour your warm organic milk and probiotic starter in a wide mouth thermos and leave it overnight. That's it! In the morning, you'll have the most nutritious diabetes-healing yogurt for your breakfast, smoothies, sauces and desserts.

DIABETES HEALING RECIPE: YOGURT

Seafood Bisque Topped with Crispy Onions
Serves: 4 to 6 servings
Prep. Time: 30 minutes

Lower your triglycerides and reduce inflammation with diabetes-healing salmon. Omega-3 rich fish helps control glucose and reduces insulin resistance. Try this healing version of rich creamy seafood bisque and don't have a moment of guilt.

INGREDIENTS:

1 tablespoon unsalted butter

4 oz. raw shrimp, peeled, deveined and chopped

1 can (3-4 oz.) wild-caught salmon

½ medium onion, chopped

2 cloves garlic, minced

2 cups lowfat milk

1 cup lowfat yogurt

GARNISH:

4 to 6 tablespoons onion, chopped

4 whole shrimp, peeled and deveined

2 teaspoons pure olive oil

INSTRUCTIONS:

1. Preheat the oven to 450 degrees F.

2. In a medium sauce pan heat the butter on medium heat and sauté the onion and garlic for 2 to 3 minutes. Add the shrimp and sauté for 2 to 3 minutes more.

3. Add the salmon and milk and bring to a simmer. Cook for 10 to 15 minutes.

4. Toss the onions in 1 teaspoon of the olive oil and spread them in a single layer on a large baking sheet. Bake for 10 to 15 minutes or until dark and crispy.

5. Transfer the soup to a blender and mix until smooth. Strain through a fine sieve or chinois and pour back into the pan.

6. Stir in the yogurt and reheat.

7. Toss the shrimp with the other teaspoon of olive oil and bake for 3 to 5 minutes or until cooked through.

8. Serve the soup with the crispy onions and whole shrimp on top.

TIPS AND NOTES:

Try minced scallops as well as shrimp for an extra depth of flavor.

> **NUTRITION FACTS:** *Calories 216.1, Total Fat 8.9g, Sat. Fat 3g, Cholesterol 66.1mg, Sodium 133.9mg, Carbs 14.4g, Fiber 0.6g, Sugars 9.6g, Protein 18.4g*

GRAPEFRUIT IS GREAT FOR DIABETES

eGL (1 cup) = 7

GRAPEFRUIT IS A GREAT FRUIT in the Diabetes Healing Diet because of its low GL and abundant store of antioxidants like vitamin C and *lycopene*, which boost immunity and prevent cell damage. Grapefruit is also rich in pectin, an enzyme that helps control blood sugar.

Grapefruit is packed with antioxidants, which combat the damage free radicals cause to cells and organs. One grapefruit supplies over 78% of the recommended daily amount of the powerful antioxidant vitamin C. Pink grapefruits are also loaded with another powerful antioxidant, lycopene, which accounts for its rosy color.

Both vitamin C and lycopene boost immunity and prevent free radical damage than can trigger aging, high cholesterol, diabetes and diabetic complications such as cardiovascular disease. Researchers from Hebrew University's Hadassah Medical School, who performed studies on the health benefits of grapefruit, found that eating just one red grapefruit a day helped reduce heart-damaging cholesterol and triglycerides by 17% (white grapefruit came in at 15%).

Grapefruits are also rich in *pectin*, an enzyme that helps moderate wild swings in glucose levels by binding to carbohydrates and slowing their digestion in the bloodstream. Pectin also helps sensitize your cells to insulin and aids in its uptake by producing insulin-receptors on the cells. These insulin-receptors function as a kind of "doorway" that makes it easier for insulin to do its two-fold job: removing glucose from the blood and ushering it into the cells where it's needed for the body's essential fuel.

The pectin in grapefruit also helps prevent blood vessels from clogging up with cholesterol, putting a person with diabetes at risk for cardiovascular disease, as well as poor circulation, loss of feeling and a reduced ability to heal from wounds, which can lead to gangrene and amputation. In a study conducted at the University of Florida, the pectin in grapefruit was found to reduce LDL ("bad") cholesterol by over 10%.

Grapefruit and other citrus are rich in *flavonoids* that help the liver burn up surplus fats instead of allowing them to accumulate in the body. This is great news for people with diabetes, who must be careful about weight gain. UK researchers who conducted a study on 100 obese adults found that those who ate a grapefruit or drank grapefruit juice every day for three months were able to lose *six times* as much weight as those who did not. Eating grapefruit reduces levels of insulin and glucose, because the enzymes in grapefruit change how the body metabolizes fat.

Even grapefruit peel helps control blood sugar. Florida scientists report that citrus peels contain *emulin*, a compound that mimics the action of insulin and helps stabilize the amount of blood sugar in your bloodstream. Researchers at the University of Hawaii found that citrus peel protects against cardiovascular disease and inflammatory disorders such as *insulin resistance* and obesity by reducing the amount of carbohydrates absorbed after meals, speeding the removal of excess glucose from the bloodstream and increasing the sensitivity of insulin receptors. The next time you make a pot of tea, consider adding some chopped citrus peel for extra zing.

Eating half a grapefruit along with a bowl of cereal or some toast has long been the standard for a low-calorie breakfast. But grapefruit also makes a surprisingly sweet addition to salad greens. For a healthy green smoothie, blend up sections of grapefruit with fresh lettuce, parsley, sunflower sprouts, mint and other fresh greens. Avoid commercial grapefruit juice that has been concentrated or loaded with extra sugar because that will spike your glucose levels. To keep your weight down, remember to pay attention to portions, as well.

NUTS HELP CRACK DIABETES

eGL (1 ounce) = 0-5

NUTS ARE A SMART CHOICE for people with diabetes, thanks to their abundant healthy fats, vitamins and minerals that help reduce the risk of diabetes and keep it under control. Almonds are particularly beneficial, because they're both high in protein and low on the Glycemic Index (GI).

A Harvard study of 83,000 women conducted over 16 years found that those who frequently ate peanuts and tree nuts—almonds, walnuts, pecans, pistachios, cashews, macadamia, hazelnuts, Brazil nuts and pine nuts—reduced their risk of developing diabetes by an amazing 27% compared to those who rarely ate them. Those who ate at least two tablespoons of peanut butter more than five times a week were 20% less likely to develop type 2 diabetes or cardiovascular disease than those who did not. And none of the women who ate nuts had any significant change in their weight. In fact, those who ate the most nuts tended to weigh a little less!

Almonds keep your blood sugar stable. According to a study published in *Metabolism*, not only do almonds have a low GI, which means they enter the bloodstream slowly, and actually help lower the GI of the entire meal (even when the meal is a refined carbohydrate such as white bread).

Another almond study published in the *Journal of Nutrition* found that the high antioxidant content of almonds—particularly vitamin E—helps scavenge *free radicals* that result from chronically high glucose levels. Twenty different *flavonoids* in almond skin, including *catechin* (found in green tea) and *naringenin* (found in grapefruit) join up with vitamin E in the meat of the almond to double the antioxidant power. Antioxidants scavenge free radicals and help prevent the oxidative damage they do to blood vessels, which leads to *inflammation*, *metabolic syndrome* and diabetes.

Even the nut's skin is good for you. According to a study published in the *Journal of Nutrition*, researchers found that although almond skin by itself boosted the *oxidation* resistance of LDL (bad) cholesterol by 18%, when added to the almond meat, that resistance topped 52%! A quarter cup of almonds contains almost 45% of your daily nutritional value for vitamin E.

We usually think of nuts as being too high in fat and calories for a weight loss diet. Surprisingly, almonds and other nuts help you lose weight. A study published in the *International Journal of Obesity and Related Metabolic Disorders* found those who ate almonds in a low-calorie diet for six months were able to reduce their weight by 11% and their waistlines by 9%. In addition, 96% of those in the study who had Type-1 diabetes were able to reduce their need for diabetes medication. In a similar Spanish study involving 8,865 adults, those who ate nuts at least two times per week were 31% less likely to gain weight than those who seldom ate nuts.

Weight loss is ultimately about eating the right amount and kind of fats. The *monounsaturated fats* in almonds help lower LDL (bad) cholesterol and reduce the risk for cardiovascular disease, for which people with diabetes are at risk. According to a study published in the *British Journal of Nutrition*, eating almonds instead of other fats reduced LDL cholesterol from 8 to 12%.

Minerals in nuts protect your heart. Almonds are high in magnesium, which helps the blood flow more easily; a deficiency in magnesium can lead to free radical damage to the heart. A quarter cup of almonds contains almost 25% of your daily nutritional value for magnesium. Almonds are also high in manganese, which helps protect against the oxidation of LDL (bad) cholesterol, preventing the buildup of plaque in the arteries, which can lead to atherosclerosis, cardiovascular disease and stroke. A quarter cup of almonds provides 45% of your daily nutritional value for manganese.

Other nuts are great for diabetes, too. Walnuts help prevent cardiovascular complications. In a 6-month study published in *Diabetes Care*, eating walnuts was linked to a significant increase in the ratio of HDL to total cholesterol and a 10% reduction in LDL cholesterol. Walnuts are not only exceptionally high in omega-3 essential fatty acids; they also have the lowest ratio of omega-6 to omega-3 of any nut (4.2:1; the second best is macadamia at 6.3:1). Eating a diet rich in omega-3s helps prevent blood clotting and plaque build-up that can lead to atherosclerosis. Omega-3s also improve the radio of HDL (good) cholesterol to LDL (bad) cholesterol and reduce inflammation.

And according to a Spanish study of high cholesterol adults, those who ate walnuts were able to reduce their total cholesterol by 4.4-7.4% and their LDL (bad) cholesterol by 6.4-10%. A quarter cup of walnuts provides an astonishing 90.8% of your daily nutritional value of omega-3s.

Walnuts keep your heart healthy, and that's critical for diabetics who often suffer from heart complications. According to a study published in the *British Journal of Nutrition*, walnuts, pecans and chestnuts are exceptionally high in antioxidants, which can lower the risk for coronary heart disease that often results from having diabetes. In a study published in *Phytochemistry,* researchers identified 16 different antioxidant polyphenols in walnuts they describe as "remarkable." Four large studies—the Adventist Health Study, Iowa Women's Study, Nurses' Health Study and the Physician's Study—found that those who ate nuts at least 4 times a week lowered their risk for coronary heart disease by an amazing 37%.

Peanuts are technically a legume, not a nut, but they are rich in diabetes-healing fats. They contain oleic acid, the same healthy fat found in olive oil; they are also high in vitamin E and other powerful antioxidants. A study published in the journal *Food Chemistry* found that peanuts contain high concentrations of an antioxidant polyphenol called p-coumaric acid, and slow roasting (170 degrees for 20 minutes) can increase that content by 22%.

Peanuts are also high in the flavonoid *resveratrol*, an antioxidant found in red grapes and red wine linked to the "French Paradox"—which found that eating a diet high in certain fats, the way the French do, can actually benefit your heart. According to a study published in the *Journal of Agricultural and Food Chemistry*, resveratrol improves blood flow to the brain by as much as 30%, thus significantly reducing the risk of stroke, which people with diabetes must guard against.

Be careful how you store peanuts because they are susceptible to mold and fungus, including one that is a known carcinogen. To discourage fungal growth and to prevent nuts from going rancid, store raw peanuts—and all nuts—in the refrigerator. Avoid the "bulk bins" for nuts unless you are sure they are emptied and cleaned frequently, and stick to organic, raw or dry roasted, and lightly salted or salt-free nuts.

High in calories due to their healthy fat content, nuts are best enjoyed in small quantities. Try a handful or two for a midday snack, and stick to raw or lightly roasted nuts without added salt, sugar, oils or extra seasonings. Almond butter on whole grain toast makes a satisfying high-protein breakfast; add grapefruit for extra fiber and extra diabetes protection…and enjoy a smart start to your day.

DIABETES HEALING RECIPE: NUTS

Romaine Salad with Curried Nuts, Roasted Sweet Potato and Ginger Coconut Dressing
Serves: 4
Prep. Time: 45 minutes

Here is a salad that is filling enough for a full winter meal. It is healthy, packed with flavor, vitamins and spice to kick up any night of the week. The coconut in the dressing adds a special cooling creamy touch.

INGREDIENTS:

SALAD:

1 head romaine, washed and torn

1 large sweet potato, peeled and diced

2 green onions, sliced

NUTS:

½ cup nuts (cashews, peanuts, almonds, walnuts)

1 tablespoon pure olive oil

1 tablespoon yellow curry powder

¼ teaspoon garlic powder

¼ teaspoon onion powder

DRESSING:

2 tablespoons fresh ginger, minced

2 cloves garlic, minced

½ cup low-fat yogurt

2 tablespoons grapefruit juice

1 tablespoon low-fat coconut milk

INSTRUCTIONS:

1. To make the dressing, combine all ingredients in a bowl and whisk. Set aside.
2. Preheat the oven to 350 degrees F and bake the sweet potatoes for 25 to 35 minutes or until fork tender.
3. Chill completely and mix with the romaine and green onions.
4. Toss the nuts with the olive oil and bake on a cookie sheet for 5 to 7 minutes or until golden. Watch carefully so as not to burn them.
5. Combine the spice mixture and toss in a bowl with the nuts.
6. Cool and sprinkle over the salad with the dressing.

NUTRITION FACTS: *Calories 219.7, Total Fat 13g, Sat. Fat 1.4g, Cholesterol 0mg, Sodium 51.5mg, Carbs 22.5g, Fiber 5.9g, Sugars 5.4g, Protein 6.4g*

CURRY COMBATS DIABETES

eGL (1 ounce) = 3

CURRY, A MAINSTAY OF ASIAN CUISINE, is a diabetes-fighting powerhouse, thanks to its spice content. Several spices that make up traditional curries—including turmeric, cinnamon, fenugreek, cilantro, chili and ginger—all of which combat diabetes because they help reduce inflammation and insulin resistance, repair and prevent the damage done by free radicals and slow the metabolism of glucose in the bloodstream.

Turmeric gets the gold star when it comes to helping heal many diseases, especially diabetes. The key ingredient in turmeric that accounts for curry's characteristic golden glow is *curcumin* (not to be confused with cumin). Researchers at Columbia University have found that curcumin is a powerful anti-inflammatory (and remember, chronic inflammation plays a big role in developing *metabolic syndrome*, the precursor to type 2 diabetes.)

Turmeric also reduces insulin resistance and lowers cholesterol. The curcumin in turmeric also helps reduce insulin resistance, which in turn lowers excess glucose levels in the bloodstream. Curcumin is a powerful antioxidant, important for combating the damage free radicals cause to blood vessels over time. Curcumin also helps prevent cholesterol from being oxidized in the body, which is important because oxidized cholesterol damages blood vessels, builds up plaque and leads to diabetic complications such as heart disease and stroke. An Indian study found that those who ate curcumin regularly were able to drop their levels of oxidized cholesterol by 33% and their total cholesterol by 11%. At the same time, HDL (good) cholesterol increased by 29%. Curcumin also helps heal wounds, which are of concern for people with diabetes.

Cinnamon in curry powder helps insulin response by lowering glucose levels and improving your body's ability to take in insulin. Scientists at the Human Nutrition Research Center under the USDA found that a compound in cinnamon makes cells more sensitive and responsive to insulin by promoting one enzyme that helps this process, and by curbing another that blocks it.

Cinnamon also helps lower high triglyceride and cholesterol levels, two key components of metabolic syndrome, which often leads to diabetes. In a study published in *Diabetes Care*, people with type 2 diabetes who ate half a teaspoon of cinnamon daily reduced their blood sugar levels by 18–29%, triglycerides by 23–30%, LDL cholesterol by 7–27% and total cholesterol by 12–26%.

Fenugreek, another curry ingredient, helps control and lower glucose levels by curbing insulin resistance. Fenugreek helps increase the number of insulin receptors in red blood cells, thus helping cells absorb glucose from the bloodstream. Fenugreek is also a rich source of dietary fiber that helps delay the absorption of glucose. This slightly mucilaginous fiber helps reduce fat absorption, which helps protect against obesity and metabolic syndrome. In a 6-month study of people with type 2 diabetes published in *Nutrition Research*, those who ate fenugreek seed twice daily were able to decrease their glucose levels by almost 25%.

Fenugreek contains many antioxidant and anti-inflammatory compounds that help reduce the clumping of platelets, which can lead to heart disease and stroke, two diseases for which people with diabetes are at greater risk. An Indian study found that fenugreek lowers blood sugar and substantially decreases levels of total cholesterol and triglycerides without decreasing HDL (good) cholesterol.

Also known as coriander or Chinese parsley, cilantro is a potent curry spice that's beneficial for people with diabetes. Cilantro helps reduce blood sugar levels by promoting the release of insulin needed to usher glucose into the cells. Both the fresh leaves and seeds of cilantro are high in phytonutrients, flavonoids and polyphenols, including quercetin, which protects against cardiovascular disease and the eye problems associated with diabetes, especially retinopathy.

Cilantro contains powerful antioxidants that combat free radicals and help reverse the damage they do over time to blood vessels. Chlorogenic acid (also present in coffee, red wine and chocolate) helps slow the release of glucose after eating. Beta-carotene helps stop LDL (bad) cholesterol from forming into arterial plaques which can lead to diabetic complications like cardiovascular disease and stroke. Both Japanese and German researchers have also confirmed the presence of anti-inflammatories in the essential oils of cilantro.

Cilantro does even more: Indian research has found that cilantro helps reduce cholesterol and triglycerides. According to USDA scientists, cilantro also eases digestion. Just two teaspoons of coriander seeds contains almost 6% of your daily nutritional value for dietary fiber.

Diabetes compromises your ability to naturally detoxify, so cilantro's cleansing properties are especially useful. Japanese research has found that cilantro helps clear up infections, a risk for people with diabetes. Cilantro is also an excellent (and inexpensive) plant remedy for removing or chelating heavy metals such as mercury from the body. A Japanese study on treating eye infections accidentally discovered that cilantro leaves speed the body's excretion of mercury, lead and aluminum. And cilantro has the ability to kill *salmonella* bacteria; in fact, a study published by the *Journal of Agricultural and Food Chemistry* found that cilantro leaves and seeds have an antibacterial compound called *dodecenal* that tested twice as powerful as the most commonly used antibiotic for killing salmonella.

Our next curry ingredient, chili pepper, lowers blood sugar and protects the heart. The main active compound in all chili peppers, from cayenne to jalapeño, is capsaicin, which also gives curry its heat. According to an Australian study published in the *American Journal of Clinical Nutrition*, eating a hot curry laced with chili peppers helps lower your glucose levels while supporting the liver and pancreas.

The antioxidants in capsaicin help combat free radicals and fight inflammation, too. In a study of 27 adults, eating fresh chilis was found to minimize the damaging oxidation of blood fats due to free radicals. Arthritis sufferers know that capsaicin cream is an effective pain reliever to rub on their sore joints. But by helping to lower blood cholesterol and triglycerides, capsaicin also helps prevent platelet clumping that can lead to diabetic complications such as heart attack and stroke. Capsaicin is also effective in treating sensory nerve disorders, such as that found in diabetic neuropathy.

Chilis are high in vitamin C and carotenoids, which both improve insulin regulation. Two teaspoons of chili peppers provide 6% of your daily value for vitamin C and 10% of vitamin A, both of which help boost immunity (often comprised by diabetes). Chilis also help you lose weight, because the heat you feel after eating them takes energy to produce and that means calories burned.

Ginger is a spicy curry flavor, and it's also anti-inflammatory because of compounds called gingerols. A study published in *Life Sciences* found that gingerols inhibit the production of nitric oxide that quickly forms a very damaging free radical called *peroxynitrite*.

Ginger also boosts the immune system and helps soothe the digestive system. This is important for people with diabetes because elevated blood sugar tends to impair digestion and lead to gastrointestinal complications. In a study published in the *Journal of Pharmacology and Experimental Therapeutics*, ginger was found to reduce the negative effect of high blood sugar on the stomach's rhythm and rate of emptying. The researchers concluded that while bringing blood sugar down is the most important thing people with diabetes can do, eating ginger-rich foods such as curries might help improve their digestion while they do so.

Be adventurous. Many different curry dishes are standard fare at Indian restaurants, which are ubiquitous in large cities. Prepared curry dishes also appear with regularity in natural food stores, either frozen or refrigerated. But you can also add the individual spices to a wide array of common meals for some extra healing power. For instance, cinnamon easily tops off yogurt and fresh fruit. Season steamed vegetables with turmeric and add fenugreek to roast chicken or other meats.

Try your hand at Indian cooking. Mastering the art of Indian cuisine does not have to be intimidating. Start by adding typical curry spices into your daily menus. Ginger is a perfect healing companion to baked squash, or grated into hot water and lemon juice for a soothing tea. Chili powder can be added to everything from egg salad to brown rice, and cilantro adds a lively kick to salads and lightly steamed greens. Once you're familiar with the individual spices and flavors, browse through some Indian cookbooks at your local bookstore, set aside an afternoon, and try your hand at a simple curry for maximum healing benefits.

DIABETES HEALING RECIPE: CURRY

Curried Vegetable Gratin with Broccoli Cauliflower, Carrot and Tomato
Serves: 6 to 8
Prep. Time: 30 minutes

INGREDIENTS:

1 small head broccoli, cut into florets

1 small head cauliflower, cut into florets

2 teaspoons coconut oil

½ medium onion, diced

3 cloves garlic, minced

1 large carrot, peeled and large diced

1 tablespoon ginger, minced

2 medium tomatoes, seeded and large diced

3 tablespoons red curry paste

¼ cup low fat yogurt

½ cup water or low sodium vegetable broth

3 tablespoons lowfat (lite) coconut milk

TOPPING:

¼ cup whole wheat breadcrumbs

1 tablespoon melted butter

1 tablespoon red chili paste

INSTRUCTIONS:

1. Preheat oven to 400 degrees.
2. Blanch broccoli and cauliflower in boiling water for 3 minutes.

3. In a large wok or skillet, heat the coconut oil on medium heat. Add the onion, garlic, carrot, and ginger and sauté for 3 to 4 minutes stirring constantly. Add the 3 tablespoons red chili paste and stir to combine.

4. Combine broccoli, cauliflower, tomato, carrot-onion-curry mixture, yogurt, broth, and coconut milk in a bowl and mix well.

5. In a separate bowl, combine breadcrumbs, butter, and chili paste.

6. Place vegetable mixture in a shallow casserole dish, top with breadcrumb mixture, and bake for 10 to 15 minutes.

NUTRITION FACTS: *Calories 95.3, Total Fat 3.9g, Sat. Fat 2.3g, Cholesterol 4.5mg, Sodium 386.8mg, Carbs 12.7g, Fiber 2.5g, Sugars 2.9g, Protein 2.8g*

WHOLE GRAINS PREVENT BLOOD SUGAR SPIKES

eGL (1 slice multigrain bread) = 5

WHOLE GRAINS ARE A SUPERIOR SUPERFOOD for managing and healing your diabetes. Because whole grains haven't been refined or milled like white flour or white rice, they still contain their essential nutrients and fiber, crucial for stabilizing blood sugar levels and controlling your weight. Whole grains are *complex carbohydrates*, which still have their beneficial fiber or nutrients intact. A Harvard Medical Study found that replacing just a few refined carbs (such as white bread, white rice or sugary breakfast cereals) with low-calorie complex carbs, (whole grain bread, brown rice or oatmeal) reduces the risk of diabetes by 40%.

Whole grains rank very low on the Glycemic Index (GI) and thus are slow to enter the bloodstream. This is especially important for people with diabetes, who need to prevent a rush of blood sugar. Eating foods with a high GI, such as most refined carbs, causes blood sugar to spike and requires extra insulin to digest it. Generally speaking, "white foods" such as white bread, white pasta, white rice and white potatoes, have high GI scores. Foods with low GI scores, such as oat bran and barley, are also high in fiber and cause only a slight rise in blood sugars. That makes them ideal foods for glucose control. It's safe to assume that the least-processed foods, which appear closest to their natural state, have lower GI scores than processed ones.

Whole grains also help cells overcome insulin resistance. Insulin resistance, a precursor to full blown diabetes, occurs when your body no longer responds to the insulin being secreted by the pancreas. Greater amounts of insulin are then required to manage the glucose in your bloodstream. The more responsive your cells are to insulin, the better they are able to metabolize glucose, and the less likely you will be to develop diabetes. Whole grains require less insulin to digest, which helps prevent the toxic buildup of excess glucose in the bloodstream.

Whole grains can also lower your risk of complications. According to a 10-year Harvard Medical School study on 75,000 women, 97% who ate whole grains regularly were able to escape diabetes entirely. A similar 8-year study by the Black Women's Health Study on 59,000 African-American women (a population twice as likely to develop diabetes as white women) came to a similar conclusion. Eating whole grains such as wheat, oats, barley, rye, wild rice and brown rice helps prevent dangerous swings in blood sugar levels. Managing your diabetes by maintaining balance in your blood sugar means less risk of developing more serious complications down the road.

Whole grains are loaded with fiber, making them a strong ally in the fight against weight gain and obesity, which are serious risk factors for developing diabetes or complications from diabetes. How quickly a carbohydrate is broken down into glucose depends on its overall fiber content. Since fiber slows the absorption of glucose into the bloodstream, eating foods rich in fiber helps control and stabilize glucose levels. Whole grains are high in insoluble fiber, the no-calorie roughage that fills you up and helps move waste out of your system. That's important for people with diabetes because these foods aid in weight loss, which lowers insulin resistance and allows your natural insulin to do its job. Weight loss also helps drive down high blood sugar, which can help you reduce or even eliminate the need for medications.

Soluble fiber is the fiber found in oatmeal, oat brain, seeds and beans. When digested, soluble fiber turns into a sticky gel that slows the digestion of sugars and starches, controls blood sugar spikes and traps cholesterol and other fats clogging your bloodstream. A UCLA study in which obese men were allowed to eat as much food as they wanted as long as most of it came from a high-fiber fruits, vegetables and whole grains, and who walked up to an hour daily, were able to reduce their blood sugar levels by 7%, as well lower their cholesterol by an average of 20% and ease their blood pressure.

Whole grains are healing "comfort foods" that are most beneficial when eaten moderately and consistently. Rather than packing in a big load of carbs one day and skipping them the next day, which puts your blood sugars on a wild ride, it's best to eat roughly the same amount of complex carbs every day. Portions are important too. Because of their roughage content, whole grains help you feel "full" much faster than refined or processed carbohydrates, so you won't need large platefuls to satisfy your hunger. Bite for bite, vegetables and whole grains provide more nutrients and fiber, with fewer calories, than any other food group. They are your best allies when it comes to controlling your weight and your glucose levels simultaneously.

Watch out for wheat allergies. It is estimated that one in three people are sensitive or allergic to wheat (a condition known as celiac disease), but there are many other whole grains you can turn to:

- Oats are especially high in fiber and loaded with vitamins and minerals; they also contain *saponin*, which helps the pancreas regulate insulin production.

- Brown rice is another "diabetes-buster" and is high in manganese, a critical component in antioxidant enzymes, which protect the body from damaging free radicals. Buckwheat also helps stabilize glucose levels in the blood.

- Spelt, an ancient form of wheat that some people with wheat allergies can still tolerate, is higher in protein than wheat and is also high in fiber.

- Rye, another high protein grain, also triggers a slower release of glucose into the bloodstream and is a good source of magnesium, a mineral that aids the body in metabolizing glucose.

- And let's not forget barley, which many diabetics consider the perfect grain because it is high in soluble fiber and boasts the lowest GI of all the grains.

DIABETES HEALING RECIPE: WHOLE GRAINS

Cajun Red Beans with Chicken Sausage and Quinoa
Serves: 4
Prep. Time: 30 minutes

The number-one diabetes healing superfood, beans, matches up with high-protein quinoa in this recipe to create a perfect, vitamin-packed substitute for the traditional New Orleans style beans and rice. Quinoa is a gluten-free grain with all eight essential amino acids—and beans are the best blood-sugar controller out there. Add some low-fat, all-natural chicken sausage and you can feel like it's Mardi Gras any night of the week.

INGREDIENTS:

1 tablespoon pure olive oil

2 links all natural low-fat chicken sausage, cut into ½ inch slices

½ medium onion, diced

3 cloves garlic, minced

1 carrot, chopped

1 (15 oz.) can red beans, drained and rinsed

1 cup low-sodium chicken stock

½ cup canned diced tomato

½ teaspoon cayenne powder

1 tablespoon no-salt Cajun seasoning

1 cup quinoa, cooked

INSTRUCTIONS:

1. Heat the olive oil on medium high heat and sear the sausage for 2 to 3 minutes on each side or until dark brown and crispy.

2. Remove the sausage and turn the heat down to medium. Saute the onions, garlic and carrot for 5 minutes.

3. Puree ½ cup of beans, ½ cup of stock and the tomatoes in a blender until smooth.

4. Add the tomato-bean puree, spices, sausage, remaining beans and stock to pan with sauteed vegetables, bring to a simmer, and cook for 20 to 25 minutes or until thick.

5. Serve the red beans and sausage over the quinoa.

TIPS AND NOTES:

You can turn this healthy version of a New Orleans classic into a stew by adding a few extra cups of stock, or use leftovers in a healthy low-carb tortilla wrap the next day for lunch.

NUTRITION FACTS: *Calories 327.1, Total Fat 11g, Sat. Fat 1.3g, Cholesterol 60.4mg, Sodium 313mg, Carbs 44.1g, Fiber 5.9g, Sugars 4.6g, Protein 15.9g*

LEAN MEAT ADDS CLEAN PROTEIN

eGL = 0

PROTEIN IS ESSENTIAL to build strength, keep your blood sugar balanced and provide sustained energy throughout the day. People with diabetes should include a protein source—eggs, dairy products, nuts and lean meats—with every meal for stable blood sugar and energy levels.

One of the best lean meats you can choose is grass-fed beef, which has a number of benefits to recommend its use, from its high content of healthful fats like omega-3 essential fatty acids and CLA (conjugated linoleic acid) to its low calorie count. Grass-fed beef is also high in a number of nutrients, including beta-carotene and vitamin E, and is considerably less likely than factory farmed grain-fed beef to transmit infectious bacteria such as *E. coli*. In addition, pasture-raised cattle are easier on the environment and cost less to raise than grain-fed cows.

Good fats in grass-fed beef. Grass-fed beef is high in omega-3s, an essential fatty acid which is vital for all the body's functions, including cardiovascular health, proper blood sugar balance (essential for treating diabetes or avoiding it altogether), reducing inflammation in the body—which is the cornerstone of most debilitating diseases—and lowering the risk of cancer. The brain also benefits from omega-3s: people with a diet high in omega-3s are less likely to fall victim to depression, attention deficit disorder, and Alzheimer's disease.

Omega-3s can be found in abundance in wild, cold-water fish such as wild Alaskan salmon, as well as plant sources like flaxseeds and walnuts. Pasture-raised cattle also are high in omega-3s: *two to four times higher*, in fact, than grain-fed beef, which makes grass-fed beef a superior choice for animal protein in the diet. Sixty percent of the fatty acids in grass are omega-3s, which accounts for the high level in grass-fed beef. When cattle are taken from the pasture to the feed-lot to eat corn and other grains, which are low in omega-3, their omega-3 content plummets. The longer they stay in the feedlot, the lower their omega-3 drops.

The optimal omega ratio. Grass-fed beef is also superior for its super-low ratio of omega-6 to omega-3 essential fatty acids, a very desirable 2:1. This figure is important because a high ratio has been correlated with an increased risk for cancer, cardiovascular disease, allergies, depression, obesity and auto-immune disorders. The typical American diet has a ratio of around 20:1 or higher, due to its emphasis on refined processed grain products like white breads, candy, soda pop and polyunsaturated fats used for cooking oils—all foods with a very high level of omega-6. (Grain-fed beef has a ratio of 14:1.) The lack of healthful omega-3 foods in the average diet—such as wild Alaskan salmon and flaxseed as well as grass-fed beef—to balance out the essential amount of omega-6 necessary in the diet means a population at much greater risk for a number of diseases.

Lower in saturated fat and calories, too. Grass-fed beef is also much leaner than grain-fed beef, which is specifically raised to have a high fat level, even though more and more consumers as well as medical professionals shun the high saturated fat content of the beef-centric American diet as a danger to heart health. According to the *Journal of Animal Science*, grain-fed beef has a fat content of over 8 grams per 3-ounce serving (and when was the last time you were offered a 3-ounce steak?) Grass-fed beef comes in a little over 2 grams, and white-meat chicken, long considered the leanest meat you can eat, has a little over 1 gram.

Do the math. Fat has 9 calories per gram, whereas protein has only 4. A 6-ounce steak of grass-fed beef has 100 fewer calories than a 6-ounce grain-fed steak. Add in a 2:1 omega ratio for grass-fed instead of 14:1, and you can see why the culprit in our diet is not "beef," but rather the low-quality, factory feedlot beef that wreaks havoc with our nutritional balance.

More healthful fats: CLA. Conjugated linoleic acid, or CLA, is another healthy fat with multiple benefits, including powerful cancer defense. A Finnish study found that women who had the highest levels of CLA in their diet had a 60% lower risk of breast cancer than women who had the lowest amount. French researchers measured CLA levels in breast tissue and found women with the highest CLA in their tissues had a 74% lower risk of breast cancer than those with the lowest.

Grass-fed cattle raised on pasture alone produce meat and dairy products with *three to five times more CLA* than animals on grain diets. In fact, French cheese actually has among the highest amounts of CLA to be found, which is not so surprising when you consider the French reliance on traditional pasture-raised cattle—and might also be one reason why the French have such low incidences of cancer even though their diet is high in fat. Soft French cheeses that are slightly aged have CLA levels between 5.3 and 15.8 mg/g, whereas most American-made cheese from grain-fed cattle range from 2.9 to 7.1. You don't have to go to France, of course, for this benefit: you can buy American grass-fed beef and dairy products, which are amply available at farmers markets, health food stores and online, and immediately reap the benefits of this superior protein source.

CLA also reduces fat while preserving muscle tissue, a benefit in the fight against obesity, which is a risk factor for many serious diseases and their complications. A study reported in the *Journal of Nutrition* found that approximately 3.4 grams of CLA in supplement form per day was instrumental in weight loss.

Other benefits of grass-fed beef. The meat from grass-fed cattle is *four times higher* in the powerful antioxidant vitamin E than grain-fed beef; it's even higher than the vitamin E in feedlot cattle given vitamin E supplements. Vitamin E is highly protective against free radicals and the damage caused by oxidation, which makes it a powerful ally against heart disease, cancer and other diseases. It is also involved in immune function and normal cell activity, and according to studies, appears to be most effective when taken as part of a whole food rather than isolated as a supplement, making grass-fed beef and dairy products an ideal option.

Grass-fed beef is also high in beta-carotene, B vitamins thiamin and riboflavin and the minerals calcium, magnesium and potassium, all essential nutrients for optimum health. In addition, grass-fed beef is far less likely to transmit infectious bacteria like E. coli. For one thing, the cattle are fed their natural diet in their natural surroundings: live grass growing in a pasture. That keeps the overall bacteria count low, and also prevents normally occurring bacteria from becoming acid-resistant, which would allow it to survive human digestive acids and cause illness.

In a study published in *Science*, grain-fed cattle were found to harbor 6.3 million cells of E. coli per gram, whereas grass-fed cattle had only 20,000. And the amount of acid-resistant (able to survive the human digestive process to cause illness) cells was 250,000 in grain-fed beef, but so low in grass-fed beef that it didn't even register on the graph. (Normal raw meat precautions and preparation should always be observed regardless of the source of the meat.)

Greek Meatball Sandwich with Mint Sauce
Serves: 4 servings
Prep. Time: 15 minutes

INGREDIENTS:

2 pieces low-carb pita bread, cut in half to form 4 pocket breads

FOR THE MEATBALLS:

4 oz. lean ground grass-fed bison

½ cup rolled oats

1 tablespoon (1 small) marinated Greek pepper, minced

2 kalamata olives, minced

2 green olives, minced

1 tablespoon lowfat feta cheese, crumbled

2 cloves garlic, minced

2 tablespoons onion, minced

1 egg, beaten

2 teaspoons worcestershire sauce

FOR THE SAUCE:

½ cup lowfat plain yogurt

1 tablespoon lemon juice

2 tablespoons mint, chopped

1 clove garlic, minced

GARNISH:

½ cup white cabbage, shredded

¼ cup carrot, shredded

¼ small white onion, sliced thin

INSTRUCTIONS:

1. Preheat the oven to 450 degrees F.

2. Combine all the ingredients for the meatballs in a bowl and mix gently. Form into 8 to 10 meatballs about 1 inch in diameter. Bake the meatballs on a cookie sheet for 5 to 7 minutes or until cooked through.

3. While the meatballs are baking, combine the ingredients for the sauce and mix. Also combine the vegetables and toss together.

4. Assemble the sandwiches with the vegetables in the bottom of the bread, 2 to 3 balls in each pocket and top with the mint sauce.

TIPS AND NOTES:

Instead of buying a whole jar of olives and peppers, you can get the exact amount you need from the olive bar at the local health food store. You can often get a Greek mixture that includes feta and has Zaatar spice (a traditional Greek blend) already mixed in. Add some cucumber to the mint sauce for extra freshness and crunch. These meatballs are also great as an appetizer or formed into a burger.

NUTRITION FACTS: *Calories 160.9, Total Fat 4.5g, Sat. Fat 1g, Cholesterol 65.9mg, Sodium 435.7mg, Carbs 16.7g, Fiber 3.9g, Sugars 2.8g, Protein 14.6g*

Healing Diabetes With Yoga

HEALING DIABETES WITH YOGA

Yoga is an excellent tool to use in healing diabetes. It offers both physical and emotional benefits by providing gentle physical activity at a calming, meditative pace.

YOGA FOR YOUR HEALTH

Yoga is a "mindful movement" practice that is tailor-made for people with diabetes, for both its physical effects as well as for superior stress relief. As an exercise activity, it offers muscle toning, flexibility and cardiovascular benefits at a calm and gentle no-impact pace—especially suitable for people with chronic illness. Various movements and postures (called *asanas*) serve to stimulate the organs such as the liver, kidneys and adrenal glands, which results in more effective natural detoxification within the body.

And yoga movements stimulate the *vagus* nerve, which extends from the brainstem all the way to the abdomen, carrying vital information back and forth to and from the brain. The vagus nerve is responsible for controlling the heart rate, your breathing and entire digestive system, among other important functions. Ongoing yoga practice can tone the heart, banish depression, boost your energy level and balance your hormones and blood chemistry.

HOW YOGA HEALS DIABETES

The Center for the Study of Complementary and Alternative Therapies at the University of Virginia Health Systems reviewed more than two dozen scientific studies on yoga for type 2 diabetes. Those studies revealed huge physical benefits of yoga for people with diabetes, including lowering fasting glucose and after-meal glucose by one-third, and decreasing A1C by up to 27%.

Other benefits include lowering total cholesterol by 20%, and LDL ("bad") cholesterol by up to 8%, while increasing HDL ("good") cholesterol by up to 4%. Body weight drops (up to 8%) as well, a significant benefit.

Research at Ohio State University found that regular practice of yoga can significantly lower inflammation as well. Fifty women participated in the study; half had just begun to practice yoga and the other half had been at it twice a week for two years. Blood samples were taken after yoga practice, light treadmill walking and during a stress test; all the women who did not regularly practice yoga had 41% higher levels of pro-inflammatory cytokine IL-6, a substance that increases dangerous inflammation in the body.

And keeping a regular schedule of moderate exercise such as yoga helps your body use blood sugar more effectively, serving as a sort of "active insulin." Increased physical activity pumps more blood into your muscles and puts the glucose to work as fuel. Having more efficient use of your blood sugar makes your system more responsive to insulin. As you begin to reduce fat and build muscle, your entire cardiovascular system operates more efficiently as well, reducing your risk of further illness and complications.

YOGA FOR STRESS RELIEF

But the physical benefits are only one part of the beauty of yoga. Yoga is all about balance—both outer and inner balance—and that balance is what frees you from stress. Yoga calms the mind because it requires concentrated attention, not just on the body postures but also on your breathing, and this union of breath and body results in a peaceful state of mind as well as more efficient and healthy body.

Breathe Deep, Live Long

A recent study in *PLoS One* showed that meditation and yoga can even positively effect the operation of your fight-or-flight response genes, thus reducing stress. Results demonstrated that genes that help counter oxidative stress were also turned on. The point is that "you really can battle the effects of stress with your mind," says the study's co-senior author Herbert Benson, M.D.

Another important aspect of serious yoga practice is its emphasis on mindful living. Paying close attention is not just reserved for your body and your breath during poses; it extends into your daily life in the form of mindful attention to your everyday behaviors and choices too. Such mindfulness is another key to reducing your stress load. The more you pay attention to yourself, the more control you have over your responses to stress-producing circumstances.

BEGINNING A YOGA PRACTICE

Although yoga is a 5,000-year-old practice dedicated to unity between mind, body and spirit, it was perhaps inevitable that our contemporary culture would create an opportunity for yoga to also be considered a demanding fitness activity, as well as a social and shopping opportunity. Busy yoga studios with large classes, special events and shops that sell special yoga clothes, yoga mats and various accessories has created a booming industry for some.... but also a turn-off to others who may seek a more traditional and less flashy approach.

If joining a class at your neighborhood yoga studio (and yes, they are now in every neighborhood in the country) seems a daunting prospect loaded with obligation to be able to perform perfectly while dressed in the right outfit, your best bet is to search out a private teacher for a few sessions to get you started.

A class can provide you with motivation, support and added commitment; on the other hand, learning a practice in private with individual attention may create a positive new ritual to start your day, in the privacy of your own home. Yoga "therapists" who focus on yoga for health and healing will have a better understanding of the challenges you face with diabetes; try the International Association of Yoga Therapists at *www.iayt.org* for help in finding someone in your community.

Be mindful about starting a yoga practice. Yoga for healing your diabetes ideally should be a gentle and calming experience. Leave the "power yoga" classes to others for whom exertion is not an issue. Upside-down postures that seasoned yogis use should be avoided by people with diabetes if they have retinopathy. Shoulder stands, head stands, even forward bends may increase pressure in the eyes, so it's wise to speak with your eye doctor first.

And like all of the dietary changes you've been making, you'll find that yoga does work to lower your blood sugar. If you are taking medication, you will want to continue to monitor your levels and have your meds adjusted to accommodate your newly healthy status.

It's often recommended that you not eat for several hours before practicing yoga, but again, if you are on medication, this may wreak havoc with your blood sugar and your energy levels. And if you have neuropathy or foot issues, take extra care to be safe by positioning yourself near a wall for extra support. If you can't feel your feet, you will have trouble with balance poses; it's wise also to get a pair of thick-soled shoes to protect your feet and toes against injury.

GET STARTED

You can get started right now in the comfort of your own home by trying the basic yoga postures in this booklet. Practice these 11 yoga poses at least three times a week for optimal overall health.

All you need is a non-slip yoga mat...a quiet, spacious area...some comfortable clothing... and perhaps some soothing background music. Take your time with each posture, never forcing your body into an uncomfortable position. Once in the posture, breathe deeply and relax, allowing your muscles to gently stretch. Hold each posture for 30 seconds or longer. If you feel a sharp pain, immediately discontinue the posture.

Once you feel at ease with this basic series, you may want to locate a yoga teacher or regular class so you can progress to the next level. *Namaste*. (That's a traditional Hindu greeting which means "peace to you.")

STANDING POSTURES

1. Tree Pose (Vrksasana)

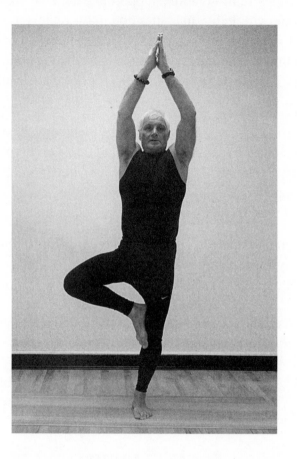

How it helps: It stretches your hips, inner thighs; while strengthening your legs, spine and core muscles.

1. Stand with your legs and feet together, hands on hips. Transfer your weight to your left foot as you bend the right knee and place the sole of the right foot on the inside of your left leg. (Beginners should start by placing their right foot at the ankle. Those with more experience may raise the right foot to the inside of the left thigh). Gently press the right foot against the left leg.

2. Bring the palms of your hands together in front of the heart in Prayer Pose. (Options include raising their hands above your head; or pressing the hands together in Prayer Pose while they are overhead.) Hold for one minute and then perform the posture on the opposite foot.

What it's good for: Tree Pose is very calming and helps focus the mind and attention. Another benefit is that it improves your sense of balance.

2. Warrior II (Virabhadrasana II)

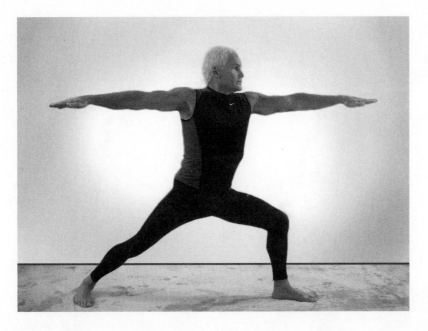

How it helps: It stretches your hips, inner thighs and chest, while strengthening your quadriceps, abdomen, shoulders.

1. While standing, step your feet about four feet apart. Turn your right foot so the toes point toward the front of your mat. Turn your left foot in approximately 30 degrees.

2. Raise your arms to shoulder height, keeping them parallel with the floor, with palms facing down. Bend your right knee so your right shin and thigh form a 90-degree angle.

3. Gently tuck your tailbone down as you draw your abdomen in. Hold for five deep breaths, breathing through your nose. Straighten the right leg and repeat on the opposite side.

What it's good for: This pose stimulates your abdominal organs, while strengthening your thighs and core muscles.

3. Chair Pose (Utkatasana)

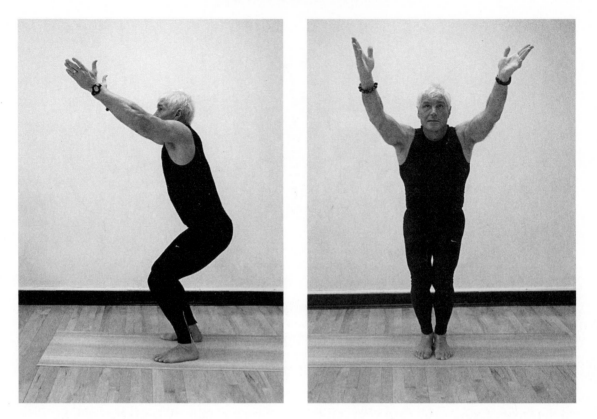

How it helps: This pose stretches your spine, while strengthening your quadriceps, ankles and back.

1. Position your feet hip-width apart, spreading your toes to create a stable base. Raise arms above your head with palms facing each another. Then bend your knees and lower your buttocks as though you were sitting into a chair.

2. Draw your abdomen in and tuck your tailbone to avoid straining your lower back. Drop all your weight into your heels, making sure your knees don't extend past your toes. Hold for five deep breaths while breathing through your nostrils. Rest for one minute and repeat one or two more times.

What it's good for: Chair Pose strengthens the quadriceps, knees and lower back, therefore protecting against injuries. It also improves posture—it is said to stimulate the abdominal organs, diaphragm and heart.

4. Garland Pose (Malasana)

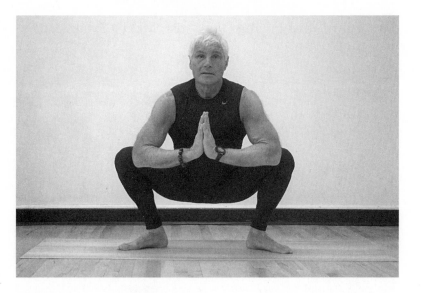

How it helps: It stretches your lower back, groin, hips and ankles.

1. Stand with feet slightly wider that hip-width. Bring the palms of your hands together in front of your heart in Prayer Pose. Turn out your toes slightly.

2. Deeply bend the knees, squatting between your legs. Keep your palms together and gently press your elbows to the insides of your knees, as it will open up the hips even more. Keep your spine long and chest open. The tension in your lower back will begin to dissolve. Hold for at least one minute.

What it's good for: Garland Pose is said to relieve gastrointestinal problems such as constipation. It's also soothing when you have menstrual cramps.

FLOOR/SITTING POSTURES

5. Downward Facing Dog (Adho Mukha Svanasana)

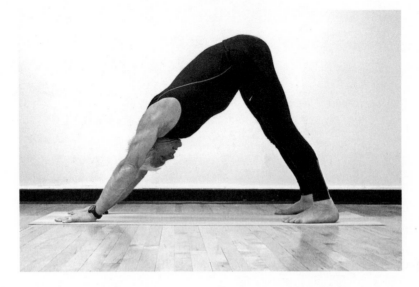

How it helps: It stretches your spine, hamstrings, gluteus and calves. It also strengthens your deltoids and triceps.

1. Start on all fours with your feet and knees hip-width apart. Position your hands about shoulder-width apart and spread your fingers wide, pressing your weight into them.

2. Lift your knees off the floor and straighten your legs. (If your hamstrings are tight, allow a gentle bend in the knees is fine.)

3. Inch your hands forward and walk your feet back to lengthen the pose. Squeeze your thighs as you press them toward the back wall, elevating your buttocks. Press your heels back and down toward the floor trying to place them on your mat.

4. Relax the head and neck and let your shoulder blades slide down your back toward your feet.

5. Breathe deeply. Hold for at least one minute.

What it's good for: This is a great upper-body strengthener. Because it's an inversion posture (meaning your hips are higher than your heart), it promotes circulation and is said to be therapeutic for high blood pressure.

6. Child's Pose (Balasana)

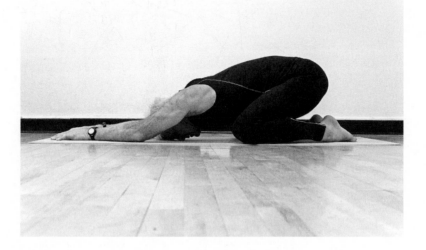

How it helps: It stretches your hips, back and quadriceps.

1. Kneel on the floor with your knees about hip-width apart, making sure your big toes touch. Sit on your heels.

2. Drop your torso between the thighs and bring your forehead to your mat. Stretch out your arms straight in front of you, with your palms down on the floor. Breathe deeply and close your eyes. Remain in this position for 30 seconds to one minute.

3. To come out of the pose, first lengthen the front torso, and then with an inhalation lift yourself up from the tailbone as it presses down and into the pelvis.

What it's good for: Balasana is a resting pose that will deeply relax you. It also opens the hips and relieves low back tightness.

7. Plank Pose

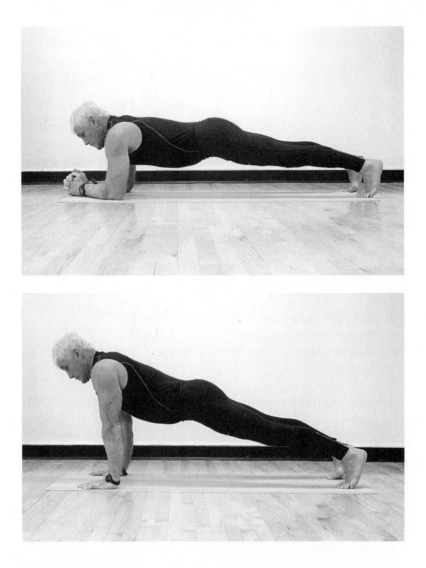

How it helps: It strengthens your arms, back, shoulders and quadriceps. Its real secret is how it tightens the abdominal muscles and builds strength in your core.

1. From the Downward-Facing Dog pose, press into the palms and bring the chest forward so that your shoulders are directly over your wrists and you are in a raised push-up position.

2. Press your heels toward the wall behind you and extend the crown of your head forward to form a straight line from the top of your head to your heels. Hold for at least one minute; but longer is better.

What it's good for: Plank is a simple but challenging way to build upper body strength because it works the major muscles in your arms, back, and core.

8. Boat Pose (Paripurna Navasana)

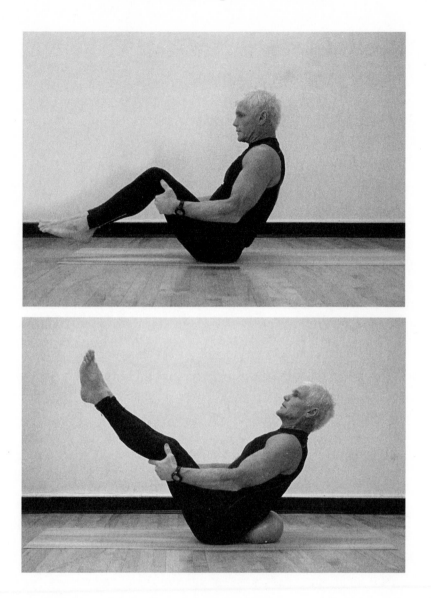

How it helps: It is especially good for strengthening your core muscles and quadriceps.

1. Sit with your knees bent and feet flat on the floor. Lean back slightly so you're balancing on your sit bones, making sure to engage your abs and core muscles to protect your lower back. Raise your legs so that your shins are parallel to the floor, with bent knees while pointing your toes. (Beginners may place a rubber ball to support the lower spine and clasp hold of their thighs. This may be enough for a while until your abs and core muscles become stronger.)

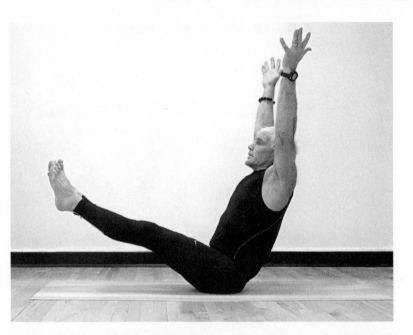

2. Extend your arms forward, parallel with the floor, palms facing each other. Keep your chest high and your core engaged and straighten your legs, trying to point your toes to the sky. Straighten arms up overhead, if possible. Hold for five to 10 breaths. Repeat three times.

   What it's good for: This is a terrific posture for strengthening your core and flattening your tummy. But it is quite challenging, so go slowly if you're just starting. Boat is also said to help relieve stress and is good for people with heart problems.

9. Half Lord of the Fishes (Ardha Matsyendrasana)

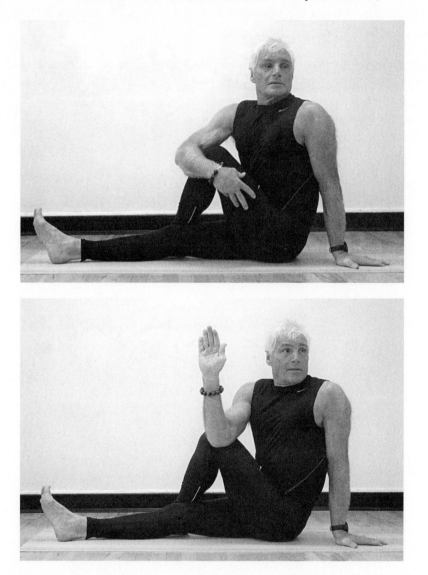

How it helps: It stretches your hips, shoulders, back and neck, while strengthening your spine.

1. Sit on the floor with legs outstretched in front of you. Place the sole of your right foot on the floor outside of the left hip, with your right knee pointing to the ceiling.

2. Bend your left knee and bring your left foot to the outside of your right hip. Place your right hand on the floor just behind your right hip. Lift your left arm to the ceiling. As you exhale, bend the left arm and place the left elbow to the outside of your right knee.

3. With each inhale, lengthen your spine and twist deeper with each exhale. Press the left elbow into your right leg to help twist the upper body more. Let your gaze look behind you. Hold for five to 10 deep breaths. Repeat on the opposite side.

What it's good for: This pose is said to improve digestion and increase blood flow to the lower GI tract. It also stimulates the liver and kidneys.

Take care: If you have an injury to your back or spine, perform this pose under the supervision of an experienced teacher.

10. Bridge Pose (Setu Bandha Sarvangasana)

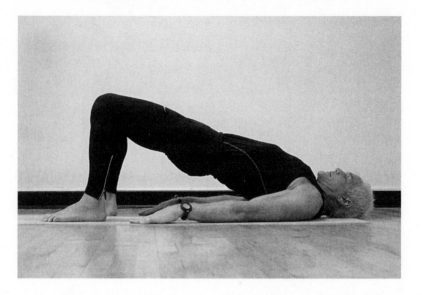

How it helps: It stretches the front of your body; while strengthening your hamstrings and gluteals.

1. Lie on your back and bend your knees so that the soles of your feet are flat on the floor about hip-width apart, with your toes pointing straight to the wall in front of you. Place your arms straight alongside your body with your palms down.

2. Press your feet into the ground as you raise hips. Allow the front of your body to slowly expand with each breath. Hold for five to 10 breaths. Repeat three times.

What it's good for: Bridge Pose opens the chest and ribcage, allowing the breath to deepen so that more oxygen will energize you. This posture is also very calming, and can relieve stress and mild depression. It is said to be therapeutic for asthma and high blood pressure.

11. Corpse Pose (Savasana)

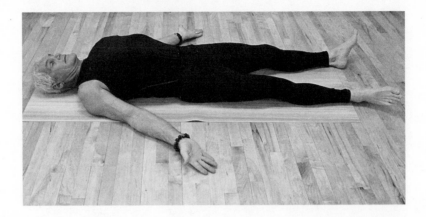

How it helps: You should always use this pose at the end of your routine.

1. Lay on your back, feet spread hip-width apart. Allow your feet to turn out. Turn the arms outward and stretch them away from the space between the shoulder blades. Rest the backs of the hands on the floor.

2. Close your eyes and breathe gently. You may want to cover yourself with a blanket to stay warm. Remain in this pose for five minutes.

3. To exit it, roll gently onto one side. With an exhalation, press your hands against the floor and lift your torso, dragging your head slowly after.

What it's good for: The deep relaxation that Corpse Pose elicits quiets stress and tension, and will bring invigorating mental energy later. You may feel as if you had fallen asleep, but this is actually a state of mind that supports the healing process.